BODY, FOOD, AND AYURVEDA

BODY, FOOD, AND AYURVEDA

The Science to Achieve a Healthy and Long Life

Arvind Yadav

DEDICATION

Mother Nature

From Whom We All Emerge

CONTENTS

ACKNOWLEDGMENTS

First of all I thank my mother and father, Rajni and Roop, who gave me life and eternal love and especially my father who, in my childhood, used to bring books during my summer vacations so that I could operate a library and rent books to friends and neighbors. I thank my brothers and sisters for their great company all throughout my life.

I thank all my Argentinian friends who blessed me with their love and strength and helped me with their best wishes and moral support, directly or indirectly.

INTRODUCTION

According to "Ayurveda," good health depends on our capacity to receive metabolic information efficiently; for example, the food we eat and digest, the manner in which we digest our thoughts and emotions or stimulate the organism due to our senses. The idea is to transmit this ancient valuable information to reach people in a very simple way in order to live a healthy life, have healthy food habits, healthy digestion and, above all, put our conscious ability in our acts to promote a happy and healthy life.

This book will guide each individual to get the basic knowledge of Ayurveda and how one can benefit from it in their daily routine. It will lead the person to see the disorders and how they can be balanced, either through diet or by changing eating habits according to one's own body–mind constitution. This book will provide valuable knowledge about the properties and uses of various ingredients which are consumed everyday so that one can decide and choose the foods which benefit their body–mind balance.

With the help of recipes given in this book, one can learn how to cook without using any kind of fat, sugar, cream, cheese and yet the food can be tasty and palatable. One can choose to cook for different disorders if already developed or to prevent them if one thinks that they have the tendency toward the same. It helps to choose the foods to be eaten in problems like cholesterol, anemia, obesity, cold, cough, etc.

Above all, the book teaches how to keep the body and mind healthy, purifying and revitalizing it periodically keeping in mind the body constitution, the *dosha* imbalance, the foods, the properties, the tastes, and the climates.

THE AYURVEDA PHILOSOPHY

It does not matter what we eat but what we digest. The most fresh and nutritive food will not have any effect on the body if the organism is not able to extract these nutrients and feed the body, that is why Ayurveda lays emphasis on the power of digesting the food and not so much on the nutritional value of the food products. Ayurvedic food need not necessarily be exotic or different in any manner, but what matters most is that it should include all the aliments cooked properly according to one's taste, with thorough knowledge of its effect on the organism. For this reason, it is very important to know the effect the food produces on our organism. Following an Ayurvedic diet will result in good health and a feeling of satisfaction and well-being. As a matter of fact, putting all the consciousness in eating the meals allows us to discover the senses, tastes, smells, colors, textures, and qualities of the food material that were ignored until now, thus enjoying the food thoroughly. At the same time, it is also recommended not to make sudden changes in the eating habits; one can incorporate Ayurvedic principles gradually and modify them according to needs of the state of health of each individual, keeping in mind the eating hours, the flavors, the textures, and the changes of the climate. Also, following the Ayurvedic cooking philosophy, each individual enjoys each meal as an act of celebration and stops eating in between the meals as this somehow manifests the anxiety and an invitation of disbalancing the *doshas*.

The most important factor to maintain equilibrium is to consume food that maintains the dominant metabolic principle or *dosha* and pacifies those that are out of balance.

Unlike western countries, Ayurveda does not account for the calorie content of the aliments. It lays emphasis on the flavors and qualities and, above all, on the efficient digestion as the nutritive value of the food product does not have any value if the organism cannot digest it properly. Basically, what matters most is to stimulate the *Agni* – the digestive power. If it does not function properly, even the most nutritive aliment will not have any effect on the physiology for not being able to be assimilated by the organism.

Ayurveda

The Indian System of Natural Cure

The life is a combination of body, mind, senses, and *atma* (spirit or the soul). They cannot be separated from each other, and at the same time cannot be neglected. From this combination ensues "*ayus*" – the span of life. Ayurveda is the knowledge of this association and of how to maintain it as long as possible.

"Ayurveda," or the science of longevity, is the Indian system of natural cure. It is known to promote a sound health, natural beauty and long life. Ayurveda, based on universal principles and a living, growing body of knowledge, is as useful today as it was in earlier centuries.

It is said that Ayurveda is as old as the world itself. It is considered to be one of the ancient systems of healing practiced by the Indian sages thousands of years ago. Its very basis is the spiritual knowledge of ancient seers of Indian and cosmic consciousness in which they lived. Into its ancient well of profound healing wisdom, some of the greatest doctors and sages over time have transforming each into one of the oldest systems which consists of theoretical basis and practical clinical applications. Its strength lies in its broad, all-encompassing view of the dynamic interrelationship between the organic and psychological processes; external factors including climates, lifestyle, and diet along with the internal psychological and spiritual condition.

Very much like various other systems of cure based on naturopathy, Ayurveda believes that disease occurs not as an arbitrary phenomenon but for definite reasons which, if correctly understood, could help to cure and, more importantly, prevent recurrence of the disease. Ideally, human beings and nature should be in perfect harmony. Disease occurs when the equilibrium between the two is disrupted. Restoration of this fundamental balance, through the use of nature and its products, is the main goal of this medical system. "The object of Ayurveda," said Susruta – a famous physician some 2600 years ago – "is the restoration of health of those who are afflicted with disease and preservation of sound health of those who are well."

Evidently, Ayurveda believes in treatment of not just the affected part but the individual as a whole. The stress is on the prevention of bodily elements and not just curing them. There are no distressing side effects of the treatment, and it has become an internationally acclaimed form of healing, rejuvenation, and healthy living.

Ayurveda considers that the body–mind organism works together to maintain a balanced health, but if one disobeys the other, the result is the disease, as somehow or the other, the error manifests its state. Therefore, it is very important to pay attention to our body needs, maintain regular routine, respect the eating hours, ensure our *Agni* works properly, as sometimes, due to various reasons, it can become weak, for example, too much physical activity, not sleeping sufficiently and properly, eating too much or very little, and so on.

Ayurveda recommends filling the stomach with two-fourths of solid food, one-fourth with liquid, and one-fourth empty, thus enabling the stomach to have sufficient space for necessary movements required for a proper and better digestion. Too much fasting is a crime against the body and can provoke a rapid increase of *ama* (toxins). Ideally, it is always better to have freshly cooked food and to avoid chemical and synthetic food products, and canned and frozen foods.

Origin and Development

Though Indian medicine has its roots in prehistoric or pre-Vedic medicine, from about 2700 B.C. to 1500 B.C., the earliest mention of medical practices is found in the Vedas, which looks back to a time around the second millennium B.C. The earliest Sanskrit treatises on Ayurveda were the *samhitas* of the great ancient physicians Bhela, Charaka, and Susruta, which date from around the Christian era. A very systematic and scientific approach, with somewhat modern ways of research and analysis, was adopted by the sages of those times, leading to the development of the system that is relevant even to this day. This encompassed not only medication but also sophisticated fields such as surgery. Sources of pre-Christian era, such as the epic Ramayana, mention remarkable feats of surgery taken place in the past. There is reference of transplantation of the eyeball. The legendary Jivaka, a famous physician of Buddha's days, is also reported to have performed remarkable cures involving deep surgery. The Indian surgeons of that era excelled in operations and their achievements in plastic surgery had no parallels anywhere in the world. Even in the 18th century, the Indian art of Rhinoplasty was studied by European surgeons.

The Science of Life

Ayurveda, with its *tridosha* or three humors system, is able to provide a complete understanding of the cause of health in terms of metabolic balance. Disease is simply understood as an imbalance between the nerve energy (*vata*), catabolic fire energy (*pitta*), and anabolic nutritive energy (*kapha*). All the food we eat has an effect on the overall balance of the respective humors. Imbalance of the *tridoshas* leads not only to impaired health but also to an impaired mental condition, because the mind's health depends on the body's health.

Ayurveda, therefore, aims to keep the three humors in equilibrium for only then can perfect health be attained and maintained. As each individual has his own particular balance or blend of these three forces, Ayurvedic treatment is person specific rather than disorder specific. The physician emphasizes a regimen of diet with the use of appropriate drugs. The age of the patient, the climate in which he lives, his cultural and social surroundings and bodily constitution need to be taken into account before offering prognosis. Touch, inspection, and interrogation are the main tools of diagnosis. In Ayurveda, diagnosis is more subjective than objective. But comprehensiveness of examination offsets any deficiencies because of the subjectivity of the diagnosis.

Ayurvedic treatment is carried out through the internal and external use of herbal medicine in a coordinated or integrated manner, as well as through surgery. Herbs are used to eliminate excesses and strengthen deficiencies. While they may possess a powerful nutritive impact on a weakened body, their primary action is to stimulate particular organic functions.

Thus, through adjustment of the diet only, Ayurveda aims to solve many health problems. Such an approach has proven effective over the centuries and as a result many of Ayurveda's healing regimens have been adapted and refined by people all over the world.

In Ayurveda, health promotion, beauty management, and healing rely on freeing the body of *ama* (toxic material resulting from incomplete digestion), restoring sound cellular nutrition, facilitating complete elimination and reestablishing balance of the *dosha*. This is gradually achieved by following an appropriate diet and lifestyle. With modern living being so inherently chaotic, such changes are quite challenging and may need considerable discipline and patience. A faster and deeper cleansing and rebalancing can be accomplished by using Ayurveda's traditional rejuvenation therapy.

Panchkarma

Ayurvedic rejuvenation therapy is the oldest scientific system for detoxification and rejuvenation of the body and mind. Although it is an ancient system, it is commonly regarded as one of the most thorough available, achieving transformative results at all levels. It rejuvenates the whole system, bringing youthfulness and strength to the body and calm openness to the mind. The combination of oleation massage, full body steam and flour scrub beautifies the skin, making it soft, smooth, and well-toned. While the specific cleansing therapies and rejuvenate tonics work on the internal body, they strengthen foundation of outer beauty and promote strength of character.

Ayurvedic rejuvenation therapy can be used as a program to improve good health, enhance natural good looks, or initiate the cure of a disorder. Traditionally undertaken as a preventive therapy at the change of seasons, both winter to spring and summer to fall, the aim is to cleanse the body not only of waste materials that may have accumulated in the body, but also excess in subtle energy or *dosha*, thereby promoting positive health longevity and balanced beauty through changing climatic condition. Rejuvenation therapy should be viewed as an integral part of ongoing self-care that helps beauty be with you throughout life. It is also an excellent, completely fresh start in the process of making health-supporting lifestyle change.

The Five Great Elements

The *rishies* (seers or sages) thousands of years ago used the theory of five elements to explain the internal and external constituents of the body. These elements are:

1. Earth: Solid state of matter;
2. Air: Gaseous state of matter;
3. Water: Liquid state of matter;
4. Fire: The force or power to transform the matter or substance into any state, that is, solid state into liquid, liquid into gas, and vice versa.
5. Ether: The place where physical existence of the state or events take place.

The Three *Doshas*

These five elements constitute the three *doshas*. The term "*dosha*" means faults or disequilibrium. The three *doshas* are:

1. *Vata*: Air force

2. *Pitta*: Fire force

3. *Kapha*: Water force

Doshas do not belong to human beings; they manifest and represent the tendencies of the cosmic universe in its whole totality. Plants, trees, flowers, animals, etc., have the same theory of *doshas* as human beings.

How the *Doshas* Work

Vata governs all that is related with the activity and movements, including the body, mind, respiration, circulation, digestion, and neuromuscular. It is responsible for transmitting information and nutrients in the organism and is the mobile force behind other *doshas*. Because of its changing nature, it is the only *dosha* which gets unbalanced much easier than the rest.

Pitta governs the metabolic and transformation functions, it is responsible for digestion, body temperature, assimilation, and coloring material of the blood and skin. It is associated with fire and water elements. Mentally, *pitta* generates new ideas and metabolizes strong emotions.

Kapha is the principal factor that provides material for maintaining the bodily structure. It is responsible for maintaining lubrication and production of respiratory system secretions; it is also responsible for physical strength rate.

The Qualities of Three *Doshas*

Vata	Pitta	Kapha
Dry	Oily	Oily
Light	Light	Heavy
Cold	Hot	Cold
Mobile	Fluid	Viscous
Irregular	Intense	Stable
Rough	Liquid	Smooth

The general characteristics of these three *doshas* to explain the bodily constituents, respectively, are as follows:

People with *Vata*-Dominating *Dosha*

- *Vata* people are very tall or very short and extremely thin people. They have difficulty in gaining weight no matter how much they eat, but their appetite, the same as all their habits, is very irregular.

- They are of dark complexion, dry skin, fine hair, and brittle fingernails; and they hardly have hair on their body.

- Their extremities tend to be cold and they hate dry and cold climates.

- *Vata* people get bored very easily, they hardly finish whatever they determine, commonly they leave everything in the middle.

- They are very sensitive to pain; they have a tendency toward rigidity, to muscular contractions, noisy articulations, gases, and constipation.

- They have a great mental agility that allows them to capture any new information quickly, but with the same speed they also tend to forget things.
- They are social, very creative, and if they get angry for something they forget it easily.
- *Vata* people are very active, they love to speak, have restless mind, as they have tendencies toward insomnia.
- They are very disordered, love to know new things, to travel, do not attach to anything, and they cannot follow any routine.
- They live accelerated, eat quickly, speak and walk quickly, and find it difficult to adapt to other rhythms much calmer than theirs.
- They are very enthusiastic, but also unstable and anxious; hence, they find it difficult to finish a project, since they change their ideas every now and then and at the same time lack patience to conclude the same.
- Soothing music, rest, warmth, meditation deep breathing, and a soft massage with lukewarm oils, or the caresses calm the increased *vata*.
- They find difficulty in making decisions, are fearful, and live worrying about small things.
- They often drift into addictions – alcohol, cigarettes, and inclosing drugs (since they always look for new sensations).
- *Vata* people spend their energy permanently since they are in movement always until the time they exhaust until they recover again.
- They can have changes of pressure and it is the *dosha* that gets unbalanced much easier than others.

People with *Pitta*-Dominating *Dosha*

- They are people of medium build, physically well formed, have an athletic body, have stable weight, hot skin, are very sensitive to the sun, with freckles or moles all over the body, and have clear and delicate eyes.

- Generally blond or redheaded, they usually get bald or gray earlier in their life. They are endowed with a very sharp intellect, an alert mind, and a great attentive capacity.

- They are highly competitive people, perfectionists, and obsessively meticulous. They follow a strict routine, are very punctual, do not like to wait and get irritated easily if there is a delay in the food.

- *Pitta* people are very ambitious, they pursue their objectives with an admirable perseverance, and usually they are successful people.

- They are very passionate in almost everything they do, that is, work, sports, and sex.

- They have an excellent digestive fire and a very good appetite; they have an efficient intestinal movement (two to three times a day).

- When they get angry, they are usually very resentful and find it difficult to forgive.

- *Pitta* people are born leaders; love to command, although it can be hard to be under the direction of an intolerant *pitta*, as they are critical and irritable.

- They can begin working from the bottom and rise up higher in much less time to be at the top compared to others.

- They are very good speakers, generally good at radio programs or TV and possess a great deductive capacity.
- They also like to climb, play tennis, or indulge in any other competitive activity.
- *Pitta* people are very intrepid and love challenges. When they face a problem, *pitta* people will not stop until the problem is solved. They are courageous and have a lot of will power and one can never see them depressed.
- They are pioneers in their fields, have a lot of will power, and when they undertake a project they do not stop until they compete it.
- Warm climate does not favor people with *pitta*; they usually perspire profusely and sometimes have a bad body odor; they generally do not use blankets in winters and they adore air conditioners.
- The cold climate balances them as well as aquatic sports.
- They lose their patience quickly and when they get angry they can be very aggressive, although they repent later, but they find it difficult to control their innate fire.
- When they are unbalanced, they incline to irritability, skin problems (rashes and acne), diarrhea, suffer from hot body, acidity, develop gastritis or ulcers, eyesight problems, become gray-headed or bald.

People with *Kapha*-Dominating *Dosha*

- *Kapha* people are big and very solid physically; possess a strong and heavy skeleton and have a lot of resistance.

- They have calm and relaxed temperament and a very stable mind.
- The hair is oily, abundant, thick, and shiny. They have a lot of corporal body hair and do not usually perspire so much.
- *Kapha* people are of white, smooth, and very soft, cold skin and with tendency to the gratitude.
- They have big and attractive eyes; the conjunctive is very white with long and dark eyelashes.
- They have a wide nose and fleshy lips. The hands are big with pale nails, very resistant, the tendons and veins are not visible, and the articulations are soft and well lubricated.
- Their nature is very sweet, are soft mannered, have lot of patience, and they hardly get angry. Tolerant enough, they forgive with ease.
- They are basically slow in all aspects: slow to walk, capture new information, digest the food, and move in general.
- They have an impressive long-term memory, although they need to be explained several times to make them understand.
- In general, they are quiet and speak when they have something important to say.
- They need a lot of incentive to undertake a project or to begin any activity, but once they start they have a lot of endurance.
- *Kapha* people have a sound sleep and find it difficult to get up in the morning. They are usually sensual and very fertile.
- They can easily gain weight and find it difficult to lose weight. They have excellent sense of pleasure

and smell. Although it is enough for them to eat small quantities but they enjoy the food so much that they usually exceed and tend to become heavy and sleepy after eating.

- Besides obesity they can have diabetes, high cholesterol, retention of liquids, and problems related with excessive mucus production, sinusitis, bronchitis, etc., their tendency to take the naps during daytime unbalance the *kapha*.
- When they face a problem, they can close up and fall in deep depression.
- They are normally good parents, loving, caring, and responsible.
- They are very attached and possessive and find it difficult to adapt to the changes. They need warm climate; they do not like cold and humid climate.

Dosha Analysis

According to *rishies*, the human body is constituted by dominating any one of these three *doshas* in combination with the rest. There are ten possible combinations:

1. Vata
2. Pitta
3. Kapha
4. Vata pitta
5. Vata kapha
6. Pitta vata
7. Pitta kapha
8. Kapha vata

9. Kapha pitta

10. Tridosha or balanced.

Normally, the human body cannot be purely *vata*, *pitta*, or *kapha* in nature, but one of these dominates the constitutional type with the rest; the body constitution is derived from constitution conditions of the parents at the time of conception, the climate or season of the year, etc. If the parents are in equilibrium according to their constitutional type during conception, the result will be a balanced healthy sibling.

To determine your own constitution, select the best possible option as accurately as you can from Table 1. Mark the selected answer and in the end sum up all the three. The *dosha* with highest marks is your main *dosha*, followed by the next. For example, if the score of your total is *vata* 11, *pitta* 17, *kapha* 7, then your constitution will be *pitta vata*, and so on.

Table 1 Know Your Constitution.

Constitution	Vata	Pitta	Kapha
Speed of work	Quick	Intermediate	Slow
Activity	Disordered	Very orderly	Orderly
Terminate what you begin	No	Yes	Sometimes
Patience	No	Irritate easily	Yes
Mental activity	Without rest	Active	Calm
Character	Changing, emotional	Perfectionist, bad humor	Calm
Memory	Short term	Good	Long term
Receptive power	Very good	Good without errors	Slow

Constitution	Vata	Pitta	Kapha
Maintain routine	No	Yes, very much	Yes
Eats a lot	Variable	Intermediate	Yes
Eats quickly	Yes	Intermediate	Slow
Digestion	Variable	Very good	Slow and heavy
Intestinal movements	Constipation	Gases	Frequent, antacid formed
Gain weight easily	No	No	Yes
Lose weight easily	Yes, a lot	Yes	No
Food temperature	Lukewarm	Cold	Hot
Uncomfortable climate	Cold	Hot	Humid
Sleep	Insomnia, interrupted	Deep	More than 8 hours
Transpiration	None	A lot with smell	Little
Under stress	Scared, anxious	Angry, decisive	Sad
Talkative	Yes	Precise	No
Form of walking	Quick	Precise	Slow
Sexual desire	Irregular	Intense	Stable
Body hair	None	Intermediate	A lot
Hair	Dry with cracks	Gray, blonde, bald	Oily, black
Skin	Dry, cold, rough	Hot, freckled	Oily, smooth
Face	Oval, unspecific	Delicate, reddish, wrinkled	Attractive

Constitution	Vata	Pitta	Kapha
Lips	Dry	Humid	Unctuous
Teeth	Irregular	Yellow	White
Tongue	Cracked	Coppery	Covered
Hands	Small or long	Medium	Big
Extremities	Lukewarm	Hot	Cold
Movements	Fast	Precise	Slow
Physical structure	Tall or short	Medium built	Large, fat
Corporal strength	Weak	Medium	Strong
Eyes	Small	Watery penetrating	Big
Eye lashes	Small, irregular	Medium	Long
Menstruation	Irregular, dolor, coagulated	Abundant, regulate	Without pain

Hours of the *Doshas*

Vata Hours

0200–0600 hours: It is the best time to wake up to start the day with vata's morning freshness, vitality, and enthusiasm.

1400–1800 hours: It is the best time to realize the mental activities, which involve creativity, imagination, studies and mental work due to *vata's* active force.

Kapha Hours

0600–1000 hours: It is the best time for exercises and strengthening work, but if one wakes up during these hours, one will be lazier and will require more strength to realize the day's activities and pass the day with the same attitude.

1800–2200 hours: It is the second best time for exercise due to active kapha's physical force.

Pitta Hours

1000–1400 hours: It is the best time to eat lunch or mid-day food as during these hours the digestive fire is at its maximum level, which makes the main meal of the day digested with ease.

2200–0200 hours: It is the best time to digest dinner and go to sleep to recover the wear and tear of body tissues during the day's activity and be ready for the next day, fresh with new force and vitality.

Climates of *Doshas*

Vata Climate

The fall and beginning of the winter, when dry and cold climate increases, the vata qualities thus making it liable to go out of balance.

Pitta Climate

The summer and end of the spring, when hot and humid climate dominates, thus increasing the *pitta*.

Kapha Climate

The spring and end of the winter, when cold and humid climate dominates, thus increasing the *kapha*.

It is advisable to keep *doshas* balanced, keeping in mind the body constitution according to the climatic conditions in order to maintain good and sound health.

Lunatic Effect on *Doshas*

New moon increases *vata*, a nice period for menstruation;
Half-moon increases *pitta*;
Full moon increases *kapha*, increases the tendencies of the retention of liquids.

Effect of Metals on *Doshas*

The gold pacifies *vata*
The silver pacifies *pitta*
The copper pacifies *kapha*

The Five Senses

All these aspects given below have their influence on *doshas* to satisfy the organism.

- The aromas of food
- The six tastes: Sweet, salt, sour, pungent, bitter, and astringent.
- The effect produced by each aliment: Heating and cooling
- The textures: Solid, semisolid, and liquid
- Colors
  Vata-pacifying colors are all shades of green color,
  Pitta-pacifying colors are all shades of blue color,
  Kapha-pacifying colors are all shades of red color.

Qualities	Vata	Pitta	Kapha
Hot	Decrease	Decrease	Decrease
Cold	Increase	Decrease	Increase
Light	Increase	Increase	Increase
Heavy	Decrease	Increase	Decrease
Dry	Increase	Increase	Decrease
Oily	Decrease	Decrease	Increase

Agni: The Sacred Fire

Agni means fire, the force, the energy, life, etc. In Ayurveda, the word "*Agni*" is referred to as digestive fire or force, emphasis is laid on stimulating the *Agni* so that digestion process works properly. Ayurveda philosophy explains that if *Agni* is well maintained, the food that is consumed digests well in time and prepares the body for next meal, absorbing all the nutrients of the foods. If *Agni* is not so strong or not functioning properly it is always better to consume cooked food, no matter, if there is little loss of nutrients during the process of cooking as emphasis is laid on proper and complete digestion and gain through remaining nutrients. One can increase or decrease *Agni* according to the state of digestive capacity, climate, eating hours, age, *doshas*, etc.

The *Agni* is considered in its normal state when:

One feels hungry in the usual eating hours and has a normal desire for food.

One feels comfortable after finishing the food.

One does not feel tired and heaviness during the digestive process.

One feels the sensation of being energetic and in good
health.

The waste products are eliminated with normal
frequency, are of normal consistency and do not
contain undigested food.

In synthesis, *Agni* is responsible for proper digestion in
gastrointestinal tract, conversion and absorption of
nutrients in the tissues providing adequate energy
and removing the waste products with ease.

Agni Related with *Doshas*

Vata Agni

People with *vata* constitution have an irregular *Agni*,
sometimes it is very high or sometimes it is low. If *Agni*
of this *dosha* is not balanced then the result will be
constipation, gases, difficulty in digesting food, etc.

Pitta Agni

People with *pitta* constitution have high *Agni*. *Pitta*
people possess a very good digestion but if *Agni* is out of
balance or in increased state, they are liable to suffer
from acidity, gastritis, ulcers, burning sensation, too
much heat, etc.

Kapha Agni

People with *kapha* constitution have low *Agni*. *Kapha*
people normally find it difficult to digest the food with
ease due to slow action of *Agni* and for that reason they
should pay special attention to stimulate their *Agni*.

They suffer from obesity, slow digestion, fatigue, laziness, etc.

AMA (Toxins)

Ama means toxins. It is an immature or unripe product, which cannot be digested. It is poisonous, toxic, greasy, bad smelling, and acts rapidly causing obstructions and heaviness in the body. There are many causes of production of *ama* in the body, one of which is weak *Agni* because of which the food remains undigested and is absorbed by the body in the form of toxins that affects the tissues, the waste channels 40 above all the *doshas* and thus inviting the diseases.

Ama forms due to inappropriate intake of food products according to one's constitution, climate, eating hours, etc. Other reasons are incorrect combinations of the foods, unripe, too much fried food, excess of food, rancid, canned and frozen food, soaked for too long in the same water, consuming heavy food without giving proper intervals in between the meals. Fasting too much, irregular eating habits, lack of exercises and walks after the foods, going to bed directly after having a meal, insomnia, taking day naps immediately after the food, worries, fear, irritation, angry, and other emotional changes are some of the reasons of accumulation of *ama*. The symptoms of the presence of *ama* are:

- Obstruction of body channels,
- Abnormal *vata* movements
- Retention of waste products

- Indigestion, heaviness in the mind and body
- Debility in the whole body
- Expectoration
- Getting tired without doing any activity
- Loss of sense and smell
- The tongue covered with a white layer indicates the presence of *ama*

The symptoms of the presence of *ama* according to *doshas*, respectively, are:

Vata Ama

The symptoms shown when *ama* is associated with *dosha vata* are obstruction of all body channels, irregular movements of gases, constipation, insomnia, arthritis, rheumatism, and nervous system problems.

Pitta Ama

The symptoms shown when *ama* is associated with *pitta* are inflammation, fever, skin problems, acne, rashes, bile troubles, bad odor, thirst, ulcers, and burning sensation.

Kapha Ama

The symptoms shown when *ama* is associated with *dosha kapha* are respiratory problems, cold, cough, mucus, sinusitis, allergies, slow digestive process, obesity, laziness, too much fatigue, and too much sleepiness.

The treatment recommended to remove the *ama* is *panchkarma* (five actions) fasting, increasing the *Agni* using various herbs and methods, balancing the *doshas* using adequate diet according to body constitution, meditation, yoga and rejuvenating the body.

The Three *Gunas*

The word "*guna*" means the state, nature, quality, desire, tendency, etc. Basically, there are three forces constituted of five great elements which determine the mental tendency of each individual namely – *sattva*, *rajas*, and *tamas*. These three states of mind are found in all human beings in different proportions, factors, aliments, and behavior. By knowing the qualities of these *gunas*, one can modify life according to the tendencies of different factors responsible for the action of each human being. The three *gunas* should be in harmony for proper functioning of mind in a healthy manner. The aliments can be transformed by cooking or processed and by the person who is responsible for cooking as the thoughts and state of the person while cooking the food is a very important factor to keep in mind.

A *sattvic* food can be transformed into *tamasic* if the person is angry or upset while cooking. In general it is very difficult in today's world to find *sattvic* aliments but it is recommendable to cultivate organic food as much as possible if not one can contact the people who dedicate in producing organic vegetables, legumes, etc. due to the growing consciousness of healthy eating.

Sattva

Sattva is considered the best and only *guna* which is responsible for proper equilibrium of the mind and the body of each individual with themselves and with others. *Sattva* means purity, light, generosity, compassion, honesty, spirituality, truth, justice, beauty, intelligence, genuine, progressive, dutiful, longevity, merciful, and harmony. *Sattva* allows having control over the senses, material world, dependence above all of the persons and objects, having faith and feeling of being devoted. It is the basis and beginning of life with virtual truth without fear and discrimination. *Sattva* people like vitalizing aliments which provide strength, health, force, joy, appetite. They prefer the food rich in flavor, nice smelling, freshly cooked, and easy to digest. The favorable foods are dates, figs, almonds, *ghee*, milk and its products, walnuts, pistachios, mostly vegetarian food, legumes, sweets, rice, wheat, honey, sugar, cashew nuts, fruits. It is important that all the food that is being consumed have its desired effect on mental organism to expand the conscience, to make the living harmonious, not to be diseased and cause disease and to eat and digest the food in adequate hours and in adequate quantities.

Rajas

Rajas is responsible for action, dissatisfaction, pain, overindulgence in sex, unstable, jealousy, ambition, dirty, meat eating, furious, irritant, terrifying others. It is also responsible for providing the movements and power of leading and organizing. It stimulates all the activities that are responsible for survival of human being in the materialistic world, leading to the satisfaction of desires like comfort, money and power in all the actions. At the same time, it is the beginning of the action providing the strength but due to its tendency of excess mental activity it ends up in debilitating the power of the discrimination. Normally, the *rajasic* foods dominate today's society and culture. *Rajas* people prefer the bitter, sour, salty, and pungent flavors which produces heaviness, sufferings, diseases, and pains. They consume very condimented foods, tea, coffee, cola drinks, mushrooms, legumes, too much fried food, fish, and poultry. They like very hot foods which dry and disequilibrate their *doshas* like onion, garlic, chilies, canned, and frozen food.

Tamas

Tamas is considered as the inertia, ignorance, darkness, pessimistic, jealousy, oversleeping, fear, egocentric, loss of memory, inactive, rancid, etc. Generally, *tamas* is related with the basics of life, instincts, corporal aspects; it is responsible for the slow actions in all aspects due to the ignorance and insufficient mental activity. The aliments preferred by the *tamas* people are bad smelling food, left overs, food kept for too long outside the refrigerator, cold stale food, impure food, and decomposed food. At the same time, *tamasic* aliments increase ignorance, ambition, criminal tendencies, inferiority complexes, and doubts. All these aliments require a great strength to digest like meats, fermented products, preserved and chemical foods, canned, packed, and the foods in bad state.

AYURVEDIC NUTRITION

The Main Food of the Day

Agni follows the rhythm of the sun and accordingly the food habits should be controlled to gain maximum benefit of the foods that are consumed and not invite diseases due to improper eating habits.

Ayurveda recommends:

The breakfast should be light in nature as the sun is in its rising stage and *Agni* is not so strong.

The lunch should be the main meal of the day as the sun is at its maximum height with utmost radiation of heat and hence the *Agni* is at its strongest point so the food that is eaten at this hour will be well digested by the body. In other words, the lunch should be only food of the day when one should eat well than the dinner or any other meal.

The dinner again should be light as the sun loses its intensity and hence *Agni* works with a slower pace. One should avoid heavy foods or meats at dinner as the body has to make an extra effort to digest the food and instead of gaining good health from food one gains diseases in the form of *ama*.

Another important factor to be taken care of is the time interval between the meals; one should give enough time for the first meal to be digested before consuming the next, otherwise none of the two digestions will be efficient resulting in the formation of *ama*. A gap of minimum 2–5 hours is recommended between the two major meals according to food intake.

One should avoid going to bed immediately after eating at night. One should have a light walk for 10–15 minutes in order to activate the digestive process and wait at least 2 hours before sleeping. At the same time, young people should avoid sleeping during the day as it lowers the metabolic rate and thus lowering the digestive process to a great extent resulting in the laziness and slow body movements especially the *kapha* people with weight problems.

Rules of Healthy Eating

- One should eat the foods sitting down and in a calm atmosphere.
- The food should be chewed thoroughly.
- Pay all the attention to the food while eating without the newspaper, the radio, the TV, etc.
- Eat according to the capacity of the appetite.
- Avoid eating if one is angry, sad, quarrelling, or in any other emotional state.
- Eat the foods according to the constitutional type, age, climate, and the state of health.

- Eat fresh and recently cooked food.
- Eat alone or in good company.
- Sip hot water in winters and at room temperature in summer, with the foods.
- Avoid cold foods and iced drinks.
- Eat lunch as the main food of the day.
- Avoid heavy food in dinner such as meats, cheese, yogurt.
- Avoid canned, bottled, and foods with artificial coloring material and conservatives.
- Preference should be given to cooked foods.
- Eat keeping proper intervals in between the meals to keep the digestion in order.
- Eat the quantity of food that is proportional to the size of stomach and not in excess.
- Fast in occasionally and not in excess.
- Keep at least 2–3 hours gap in the dinner and going to bed.
- Avoid sexual activity immediately after eating.
- Preference should be given to attain all the six flavors in each meal favoring to balance the *doshas*.
- Arrange the meals including solid foods, semisolid, liquid, and semiliquid.
- We should satisfy the five senses: colored meals, the aroma, to listen the sounds that take place when cooking and chewing, to enjoy the varied textures, and to taste the food.
- Have a light walk to facilitate the digestion.
- Try to breathe from the right nostril while consuming.

- Drink milk separately from the rest of the foods and always boil it before consuming.

- Avoid heating the honey.

- Sit down 5–10 minutes after the food giving thanks to the god for the food.

Vegetables

Vegetables are one of the most important and highly beneficial foods used since ancient times for maintenance of health and prevention of disease. They contain valuable food nutrients which helps building and repairing the body. In Ayurveda, the vegetables hold a very high place due to the curative properties discovered by *rishies* in ancient times.

Vegetables are important in maintaining the alkaline balance and, at the same time, they are valued for their high vitamin and mineral contents. They are rich in vitamins and low in calories, being light and moist they are easy to digest when cooked properly. They can be combined with almost all other foods. In Ayurveda, the vegetables are classified as light or heavy, cool or warm, and dry or oily. In most of the cases, warm vegetables tend to pacify *vata* and *kapha*, while the cool vegetables pacify *pitta*. Apart from this, their properties can be altered according to one's *dosha* by using different spices and mode of cooking.

Care should be taken while cooking vegetables as overcooking and careless storage can destroy their valuable nutrients. They are consumed in the forms of leaves, stems, roots, fruits, seeds, and flowers. Each group contributes to form a complete nutritional diet required by a human being providing the vital proteins, vitamins, carbohydrates, and minerals.

It is very essential to consume vegetables fresh in order to get maximum benefits of their qualities. Most leafy vegetables are best consumed raw in the form of salads except for *vata* people who can use it by putting more dressing to it. Care should be taken while cooking the vegetables in order to preserve all the nutrients to its maximum extent possible. Some important hints for proper cooking of vegetables are as follows:

- First of all vegetables should be washed thoroughly and cooking time adjusted according to size of the cut and the type of vegetables.

- The vegetables should be boiled with little salt in order to prevent the loss of vitamin C and B complex.

- It is much better if vegetables are covered while cooking using just the sufficient amount of water and in case of leafy vegetables one can avoid adding water because of their high moisture content.

- All the legumes should be soaked overnight to make it more digestible.

- It is advisable to scrape instead of peeling the vegetables in order to avoid loss of large amount of minerals present directly under the skin.

- One should avoid cooking in aluminum utensils as being a soft metal it is acted upon by both food acids and alkalis. The scientific explanation is that the aluminum particles being very astringent, injure the

- sensitive lining of the stomach leading to gastric irritation, digestive, and intestinal ailments.

Water

When to drink water has always been a dispute, but Ayurveda explains it clearly, considering that the water has cold and heavy properties. Thus to convert the heavy properties into the light ones, one should boil it, at the same time consuming ice cold water makes the digestive process work slow thus increasing *kapha*. The best time to drink water is during the meals but not more than a cup, as it helps in the proper digestion of the food.

Drinking water before the food increases *vata*.

Drinking water during the food in small quantities increases *pitta* which is good for digestion.

Drinking water after the food increases *kapha*, above all *kapha* people should take more care because of their water retention tendency.

Milk

Milk is considered as a complete meal as it has all the nutrients needed by the body. It is heavy and cold and has sweet postdigestive effect. It is good for all the *doshas* but *kapha* people should take in moderate amount or take fatless milk. It is always good to boil the milk to make it light and easily digestible, at the same time it can be boiled with spices like ginger, cardamom, saffron etc. in order to make it heating in nature. In western countries, the terms pasteurized and homogenized milk is very confusing for people as it gives them the idea that after these processes the milk is safe to drink but it is not so. It should not be cooked or mixed with other food or salty meals; it can be combined with sweet aliments like *ghee*, rice, wheat, almonds, walnuts, cashew nuts, pistachios, figs, dates, raisins, etc.

To replace the milk in cooking, soymilk is highly recommended, for example, making white sauce, soups, and similar other uses.

Honey

Since ancient times honey holds a high place in Indian medicine for its curative properties, a natural sweetener, provides the body instant energy or glucose as it directly goes into the blood stream like alcohol and for that reason the *vaidyas* (Ayurvedic Doctors) use to give the medicines mixed with honey. Best for *kapha*, but *vata* and *pitta* should take in moderate amounts as it is heating and drying in nature thus have a tendency of increasing *vata* and *pitta* when taken in excess.

Boiled or heated honey is very toxic and for that reason one should not cook the desserts, cookies, and sweets with honey, at the same time one should mix honey in warm beverages and not hot in temperature.

Vata-Pacifying Diet

Vegetables (fresh, cooked, and of the season)
Sweet potato, carrot, green beans, pumpkin, squash, round gourd, butter beans, water cress, cooked fennel, asparagus, artichoke, avocado, olives, beetroot, lady fingers, radish

Reduce: potato, tomato (without seeds and skin), spinach, sweet corn, capsicum, long gourd, cucumber

Avoid: mushrooms, cauliflower, lettuce, endives, radish, peas, garlic onion, cabbage, brussels, celery, eggplant, broccoli, soy sprouts

Fruits (fresh, sweet, and juicy)

Dates, damask, mango, peach, banana (very mature), plum, coconut, figs, papaya, sweet pineapple, kiwi, lemon, melon, orange, sweet lime, grapes, cherry

Reduce: the quantity of: pear, apple, and blueberry

Avoid: dry and immature fruits (especially banana) quince, pomegranate

Cereals

Rice: basmati, yamani, integral rice, wheat (well cooked)

Reduce: quinoa, rye, couscous

Avoid: corn, barley, amaranth, millet

Legumes

Mung, aduki, red lentils, tofu, kidney beans

Reduce: soya beans, *urad*, black chickpeas, and black lentils

Avoid: chickpeas, black beans, and white beans

Dairy Product

Ghee, whole milk, lassi *vata*, ricotta, cottage, shortening, cream, creamy cheeses, yogurt

Reduce: ice creams

Avoid: hard cheeses, powdered milk

Nuts

Almonds (peeled), pistachios, walnuts, cashew nuts
Reduce: sunflower seeds, safflower, sesame seeds
Avoid: peanut

Oil

Sesame, almond, sunflower, canola
Reduce: olive, soya, coconut, mustard, corn
Avoid: animal fat

Sweeteners

Cane sugar, turbinado, maple syrup, and fructose
Reduce: white sugar, honey
Avoid: heated or cooked honey, artificial sweeteners

Spices

Cumin, asafetida, basil, bay leaf, cardamom, black pepper, anisette, mustard seeds, nutmeg, cinnamon, cloves, oregano, saffron, turmeric, tamarind, vanilla, sweet pepper, curry powder, dill, fresh ginger, fennel seeds, thyme, poppy seeds
Reduce: fenugreek, mint, parsley, cayenne pepper, coriander
Avoid: garlic, onion

Drinks

Juices of papaya, orange, peach, carrot, mango, grape, aloe vera, grapefruit, damask, coconut milk, lemonade, almond milk
Reduce: banana shake, apple juice, lassi *vata* (yogurt diluted with water – sweet or salted), pear, berry, tomato (strained)
Avoid: iced drinks, soda, drinks with caffeine, alcohol

Tea

Licorice, cardamom, cinnamon, lemon, orange, fresh ginger, fennel, lavender, rose

Avoid: black tea, jasmine, coffee, and ginseng

Pitta-Pacifying Diet

Vegetables

Cucumber, asparagus, potato, sweet potato, cauliflower, lettuce, green beans, cabbage, brussels, broccoli, artichoke, endives, water cress, squash, pumpkin, sprouts, *karela*, sweet corn, mushrooms, lady fingers, avocado

Reduce: celery, spinach, boiled onion, carrot, beetroot, parsley, radish, olives

Avoid: radish, garlic, raw onion, eggplant, chili, tomato, olives in brine

Fruits

Coconut, figs, dates, apple, pear, damask, melon, sweet grapes, mango, pomegranate, sweet pineapple, cherries, quince, plums, peach

Reduce: dry fruits, orange lemon, kiwi, strawberry (sweet)

Avoid: tamarind, grapefruit sweet lime (sour), papaya

Cereals

Rice, wheat, rye

Reduce: barley, quinoa, corn, millet, amaranth, integral rice

Legumes

Chickpeas, black lentils, Aduki beans, *mung*, black beans, soya beans, tofu, green peas

Avoid: red lentils

Nuts

Sunflower seeds, coconut, pumpkin seeds

Reduce: walnuts, peeled almonds, cashew nuts, and pistachios

Avoid: peanut and any type of salted nuts

Dairy Product

Ghee, milk, shortening, *pitta* lassi, ice creams, cottage cheese, cream

Reduce: ricotta, creamy cheeses

Avoid: yogurt, hard and fermented cheeses, sour cream, and powdered milk

Oil

Coconut, soya, olive, sunflower

Reduce: sesame, almond

Avoid: mustard, corn, animal fat

Sweeteners

Maple syrup, fructose, turbinado (cane sugar)

Reduce: honey (mainly at noon), white sugar

Avoid: molasses, artificial sweeteners

Spices

Coriander, cilantro, cardamom, fennel, mint, cinnamon, turmeric, anisette, dill, licorice, saffron

Reduce: fresh ginger, nutmeg, cumin, cloves, sweet pepper, curry powder, vanilla, basil

Avoid: asafetida, salt, cayenne pepper, mustard seeds, oregano, bay leaf, fenugreek, dry ginger, onion, and chili

Drinks

Apple juice, grape, peach, pear, mango, damask, dates shakes, coconut, figs, coconut milk, *pitta* lassi, aloe, soya milk

Reduce: almond milk

Avoid: coffee, alcohol, soda, chocolate shake, tomato, grapefruit, papaya juice, orange, banana shake

Tea

Jasmine, lavender, chamomile, fennel, mint, cinnamon, licorice, rose, cardamom

Avoid: ginseng, ginger

Kapha-Pacifying Diet

Vegetables

Broccoli, cabbage, brussels, asparagus, mushrooms, artichoke, carrot, karela, pepper, cauliflower, radish, lettuce, endives, celery, beetroot, eggplant, lady fingers, spinach, peas, round gourd

Reduce: cucumber, squash, pumpkin, long gourd, potato, tomato

Avoid: sweet potato, tapioca, avocado, olives

Fruits

Dry figs, peaches, raisins, pomegranate, apple, pear, quince, damask, guava, blueberry, and dry fruits

Reduce: sweet lime, orange, kiwi, mango, lemon, strawberries, grapes, dates, tamarind, papaya, cherries

Avoid: grapefruit, fresh figs, banana, coconut, melon, pineapple, plum, and all excessively sweet or sour fruit

Cereals
Millet, rye, barley, corn
Reduce: amaranth, quinoa, rice
Avoid: wheat, rice flour

Legumes
Lentils, chickpeas, black beans, aduki beans, mung beans
Reduce: Tofu (well cooked), white beans
Avoid: Soya beans, red lentils

Nuts
Sunflower seeds, pumpkin seeds, and poppy seeds
Avoid: the rest

Dairy Product
Goat milk
Reduce: Fatless milk, *kapha* lassi, *ghee*, goat cheese, cottage cheese, and ricotta
Avoid: Yogurt, cream, shortening, cheeses, ice creams, whole milk

Oil
Small quantities of corn oil, sunflower, almond, mustard, sesame
Avoid: Olive, coconut

Sweeteners
Honey (without heating)
Reduce: Fructose (small quantities)
Avoid: White, cane sugar (turbinado), molasses, artificial sweeteners

Spices

Chili, white pepper, black pepper, cayenne pepper, fresh and powdered ginger, cloves, nutmeg, fenugreek, mustard seeds, cumin, turmeric, coriander, oregano, cardamom, licorice, basil, fennel, cinnamon, asafetida, anisette, parsley, saffron, thyme

Avoid: salt, vinegar, and miso

Drinks

Juices of apple, pear, carrot, pomegranate, blueberry, damask, aloe, karela, coconut water, coffee (decaffeinated)

Reduce: Papaya juice, mango, orange juice, sweet lime, lemonade

Avoid: Iced, soda, alcohol, milk, chocolate shake, banana shake, tomato

Tea

Chamomile, clove, cinnamon, cardamom, ginger, jasmine, rose, licorice, basil, cedron

Reduce: drinks immediately after eating (to wait 2 hours).

The Six Flavors

Ayurveda considers that there are six essential flavors that are needed by the human body to satisfy the appetite and should be present in each meal. They are as follows:

- Sweet
- Salty
- Sour

- Bitter
- Pungent
- Astringent

The six flavors are constituted by the five great elements same as the three *doshas*.

Sweet	Water and Earth
Salty	Fire and Water
Sour	Fire and Earth
Bitter	Air and Ether
Pungent	Fire and Air
Astringent	Earth and Air

Flavors	Vata	Pitta	Kapha
Sweet	Decrease	Decrease	Increase
Salty	Decrease	Increase	Increase
Sour	Decrease	Increase	Increase
Bitter	Increase	Decrease	Decrease
Astringent	Increase	Decrease	Decrease
Pungent	Increase	Increase	Decrease

Ayurveda considers that the theory of six flavors acts on the organism in a very peculiar manner. Each of these flavors have their own properties which can be light, dry, heavy, oily, hot, or cold. In this manner, it helps in determining the aliments, ease the light ones or having difficulty in the heavy ones to digest, dehydration or lubrication of the body, pacifying or stimulating effect on the three *doshas*, etc.

The Functions of the Flavors

Sweet

The sweet flavor pacifies *vata*, *pitta*, and increase *kapha*. It is responsible for the growth of all the tissues, nurturing the body and helps in the growing stage of children and adults providing strength, vigor, firmness, vitality, stability, and a robust body. It brings instant relief in the conditions of the burning sensation, thirst, and hunger.

Sweet is oily, heavy, and cold; it helps in pacifying the digestive fire.

Vata people do well with sweet flavor; it helps in restoring the physical strength, equilibrium, and stability.

Pitta people benefit the most with this flavor due to its cold nature as it pacifies the innate heat of a *pitta*.

Kapha people are the ones who have to take special care with flavor as being heavy in nature it increases *kapha*, thus causing obesity, obstructions, slow digestion, congestion, etc. At the same time, they are the ones who get tempted by this flavor than the rest.

The source of sweet flavor is all the sugars, rice, most of the dry fruits, cream, milk, *ghee*, potatoes, sweet potato, squash, meat for nonvegetarians.

Salty

A salty flavor pacifies *vata* and increases *pitta* and *kapha*; it is light, oily, heating, and with sweet postdigestive effect. It stimulates digestion and gastric juices in the mouth and intestine. This flavor is laxative in nature and helps in the smooth flow of body fluids in different circulation channels.

Vata people benefit the most and only *dosha* to handle salt with ease as it provides the light heating effect, lubrication, and regulating the digestive fire. Emotionally, it provides warmth to life.

Pitta people get disequilibrated with ease with salty flavor causing burning sensation, acidity, ulcers, and too much thirst.

Kapha people have a tendency of suffering from retention of liquids with excess of salt.

Ayurveda mentions five varieties of salt; the black salt variety is widely used medicinally mainly to reduce flatulence and gas troubles.

The sources of salt flavor are all salts, soy sauce, french fries, snacks, most of the canned foods, pickles, etc.

Sour

The sour flavor pacifies *vata* and increases *pitta* and *kapha*. It is light, oily, heating with sour postdigestive effect. The flavor sour is carminative, increases the appetite, and stimulates the secretions, digestive fire and thirst. It stabilizes the functions of the senses, clears and helps in better functioning of mind. Emotionally when the sour flavor is balanced enhances the adventurous spirit, awareness of the conscience and a sensation of the truth and realism. On the contrary, if this flavor is out of balance generates jealousy, anger, irritation, untrustworthy, and not reliable.

Vata people benefit the most with this flavor as sour flavor pacifies the *vata* to great extent. It regulates and stimulates the irregular digestive fire of *vata*; it provides strength and force to the body and calms the nervous system of an accelerated *vata* and helps in downward movement of the food.

Pitta people should take special care from this flavor as it tends to increase the *pitta* to a great extent when taken in excess causing acidity, ulcers, burning sensation, skin problems, and similar other problems.

Kapha people should also avoid an excess intake of this flavor as it creates the tendency of the liquid retention.

The source of sour flavor are all citric aliments, vinegar, cheese, tomato, pickles, alcohol, curd, lemon, orange, sweet lime, tamarind, mango, etc.

Bitter

The bitter flavor pacifies *pitta* and *kapha* and increases *vata*. It is cooling, light, and dry in nature with pungent postdigestive effect. It is one of the flavors which are used quite less due to its bitterness but it enhances the other flavors. It purifies the organism and the blood, dries the body secretions, pacifies the thirst, and is considered as an antidote for the parasites, fevers, poisoning, fainting, burns, sun stroke, etc. It helps in stimulating the appetite and increases the maternal milk. Emotionally it stimulates the intellect power, the change, memory, conscience but in excess it produces frustration and disheartedness.

Vata people should avoid this flavor because it disequilibrates this *dosha* due to its light, dry, and cold properties. It generates instability, nervous disorders, general weakness, and dries body secretions.

Pitta people benefit the most with this flavor due to its coldness thus cooling the *pitta*'s gastrointestinal tract which is always on fire.

Kapha people also benefit with this flavor despite being cold in nature as it helps in drying body secretions, losing weight, and removing the obstruction of blocked circulation channels.

The source of this flavor are all greens like spinach, endives, parsley, etc. all sprouts, turmeric, mint, coffee, tea, legumes and beans, millet, barley, etc.

Astringent

The astringent flavor pacifies *pitta* and *kapha* and increases *vata*. It is light, dry, cooling with pungent postdigestive effect. Astringent flavor is sedative, drying, constrictive, dries the internal secretions; it dries the wounds and cures ulcers. It is also beneficial in respiratory problems, congestion etc. In excess, it produces constipation, obstruction of the body channels, thirst, and digestive fluids especially the lower part obstructing feces movement. Emotionally in excess it produces fairness, insecure, introversion, and loss of interests in general.

Vata people should avoid this flavor in excess as it can disequilibrate this *dosha* easily due to its drying, light, and cooling properties, slow digestion due to its contracting effect and thus slowing and drying the bodily secretions.

Pitta people benefit with this flavor due to its cooling effect thus calming the furious *pitta*, it helps reducing the innate fire, acidity, gastritis, ulcers, fevers, and other *pitta*-related problems.

Kapha people benefit the most with this flavor as it has a pacifying effect on *kapha* due to its tendencies of drying the body fluids, retention of liquids, and helps in *kapha*-related problems.

The sources of astringent flavor are tea, coffee, pomegranate, banana, legumes, cauliflower, cabbage, spinach, and most leafy vegetables.

Pungent

The pungent flavor pacifies *kapha* to a great extent and increases *vata* and *pitta*. It is light, dry, heating with pungent postdigestive effect. This flavor reduces heat, burns excess fat, semen, mother's milk, and can even cause abortion if taken in excess. At the same time, it stimulates *Agni* the digestive fire, favors better digestion and absorption by the organism, helps in obesity, mouth purification, humidity, remove the obstructing particles, it is expectorant and dries the congestion. Emotionally, it produces passion, stimulates the movements physically and mentally and an extroverted character, in excess it produces irritating and impatient nature, aggressiveness, and intolerance.

Vata people should consume this flavor in little quantities as it favors this *dosha* in stimulating its digestive fire, but in excess it can dry the body secretions.

Pitta people should avoid this flavor as it increases the fire thus disequilibrating the *pitta* causing problems like acidity, burning sensation, skin rashes, etc.

Kapha people benefit the most with flavor as it stimulates the lazy *kapha* and equilibrate the oily, heavy, and cold properties, it activates *kapha*'s slow digestion, stops retention of liquids, and above all scrapes away the excess fat.

The sources of pungent flavor are the chilies, mustard, onion, ginger, garlic, black pepper, radish, sweet pepper, etc.

Reaction of Flavors on Emotions

Flavor	Normal	In excess
Sweet	Satisfaction	Complacence
Salty	Adventure	Jealousy
Sour	Zest	Hedonism
Bitter	Desire	Frustration
Astringent	Introversion	Insecure
Pungent	Irritable	Extroversion

Rasa (Flavor)

Flavor	Element	Properties	Increase	Decrease
Sweet	Water–earth	Cold–heavy–oily	Vata–pitta	Kapha
Salty	Fire–water	Hot–heavy–oily	Vata	Pitta–kapha
Sour	Earth–fire	Hot–heavy–oily	Vata	Pitta–kapha
Bitter	Air–ether	Cold–light–dry	Kapha–pitta	Vata
Astringent	Air–earth	Cold–light–dry	Pitta–kapha	Vata
Pungent	Fire–air	Hot–light–dry	Kapha	Pitta–vata

Vipak: The Postdigestive Effect of the Flavors

Flavor	Vipak
Sweet	Sweet
Salty	Sweet
Sour	Sour
Bitter	Pungent
Astringent	Pungent
Pungent	Pungent

Spices and Condiments

Ginger

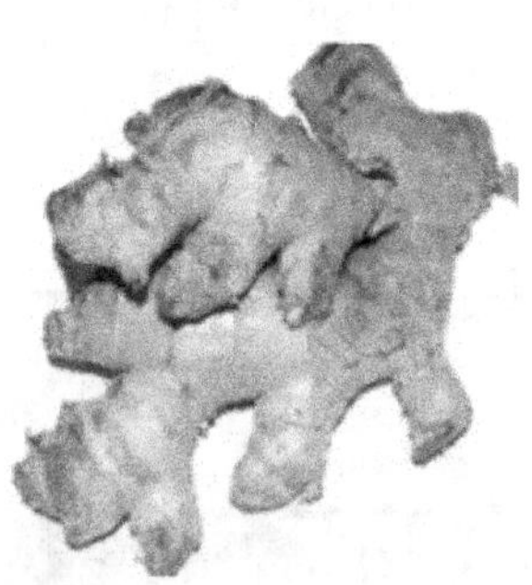

Ginger is native rhizome of Asia and broadly used in India in cuisine and as medicine. The properties differ a lot depending if it is used fresh or in dry form. Fresh ginger is heavy, dry, strong, and pungent but with sweet postdigestive effect, therefore *pitta* does not get unbalanced and all the *doshas* can use it with ease.

Fresh ginger increases the digestive fire and people with slow digestion should take ginger in form of decoction or chewing a piece half an hour before lunch and dinner. It alleviates the abdominal distension due to gases.

Dry ginger is light, oleaginous, hot, and pungent, good for *vata* and *kapha*.

Dry ginger can be applied on forehead in the form of paste to reduce headaches. It has great effect in the rheumatic conditions and in all conditions of increased *ama*. It is used as much for diarrhea as for constipation. It is beneficial in congestion, it is expectorant and anti-nausea. It promotes circulation when applied on the skin. It is also considered beneficial in vomiting, jet lag, dizziness, hemorrhoids, heart disorders, hypotension, fever, colds, and above all helps in scraping the long-seated *ama* (toxins) in the body.

Turmeric

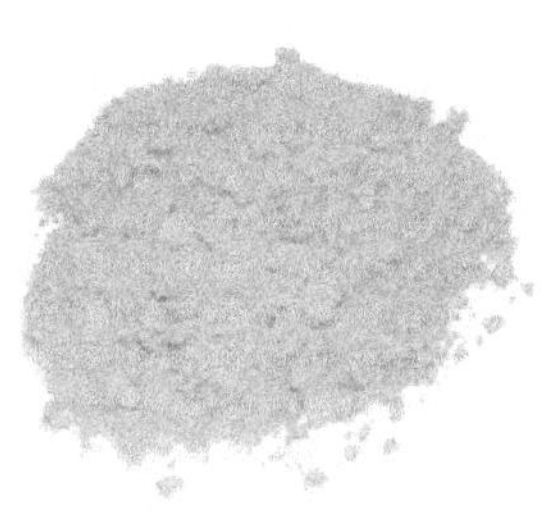

Turmeric is the native rhizome of India and South Asia. It is bitter, astringent, and pungent in nature and has hot and pungent postdigestive effect. It is light and dry and balances the three *doshas,* but when in excess it unbalances *vata* and *pitta,* can be used internally and externally, raw or cooked. Its antiseptic action has been scientifically proven; it is used on open wound, stings of insects, stops bleeding, eczemas, acne, and other skin problems. It can be used in the form of vapor for cleaning eyes, and internally it acts as a natural antibiotic. Turmeric can be taken in throat pains, cough and cold by boiling half teaspoon of turmeric with one cup of milk, and in intestinal infections a piece of the root can be chewed. It stimulates digestion and balances the intestinal fluid. It serves as a blood cleanser, is very effective in diabetic's diet, and has antiallergic properties. It is also used in amenorrhea, anemia, and blood circulation.

Cardamom

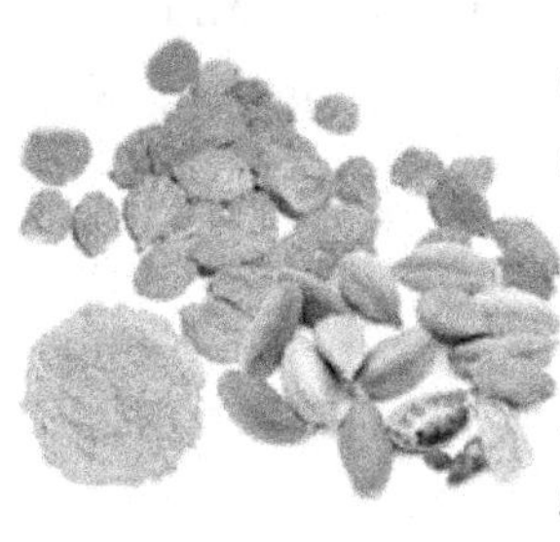

Cardamom is sweet, pungent, hot, and has a sweet postdigestive effect. It increases *Agni* and *ojas* without increasing *pitta*. All the *doshas* are at ease with cardamom. It is considered to be the safest *sattvic* digestive stimulant for all ages and removes *Ama* (toxins) from the body. It is used as carminative and reduces heat of the mind and body. It is beneficial in cases of abdominal distension, hemorrhoids, and urinary infections. It is also recommended in heart infections, asthma, cough, and as natural antacid. The Middle East culture always uses it powdered together with coffee to counteract acidity produced by caffeine and in turn gives a peculiar flavor. When added to milk or ice creams, it neutralizes mucus-forming properties. It is a good expectorant used in bronchitis, cough, asthma, and hoarseness. It stops sour regurgitation, burps, and vomits. In India, it is widely used for bad breath by chewing the seeds and used as the main ingredient in Indian desserts.

Black Pepper

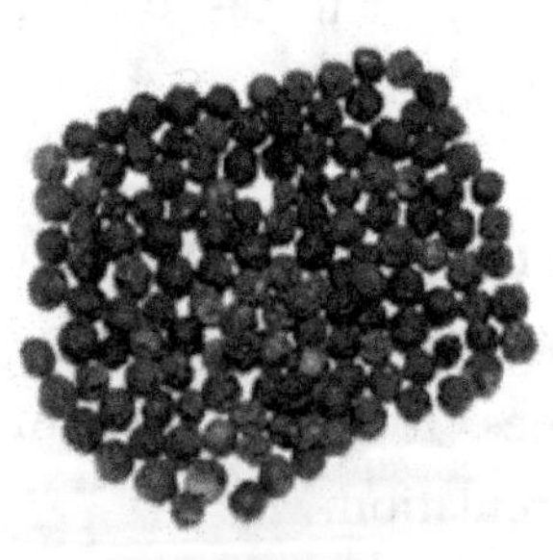

Black pepper is pungent, hot, dry, and has a pungent postdigestive effect. It pacifies *vata* and *kapha* and increases *pitta*. It is one of the digestive but strong stimulants, burning toxins and cleaning the gastrointestinal tract. In case of congestion sinuses, migraines, and even convulsions, it can be used as nasal application mixed with *ghee*. With honey, it is a good expectorant and mucus cleaner, drying secretions. In excess, it can irritate the mucus. Externally, it is good to develop and promote the suppuration. It is good to accompany raw foods and salads. It is one of the most important spices of all the cuisines of the world.

Coriander

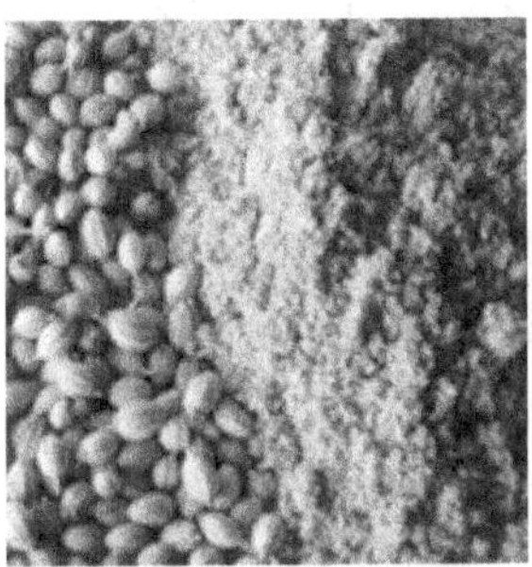

Coriander is probably native of the Mediterranean region. It is an aromatic herb of bitter, slightly pungent, and sweet and contains very little astringent flavor. Its therapeutic action is basically due to its cooling effect. The postdigestive effect is sweet. It pacifies *vata* and *kapha*. It cools *pitta* when cooling the body heat, mainly of eyes and intestines. It acts as diuretic, carminative, and stimulates the appetite. It is used in the form of decoction in fever to reduce the burning sensation and washing eyes in conjunctivitis. Its infusion is useful in urinary problems and hemorrhoid conditions. It is also considered beneficial in burning urethra, sore throat, vomiting, allergies, and hay fever.

Cilantro (*Hara Dhania*)

The cilantro leaf has a cooling effect and it is used to pacify *pitta.* Its juice neutralizes the poison of insects and spiders' sting. It is effective in allergies, cutaneous eruptions, rashes, and fever. Externally, it can also be used in stings and inflammation conditions.

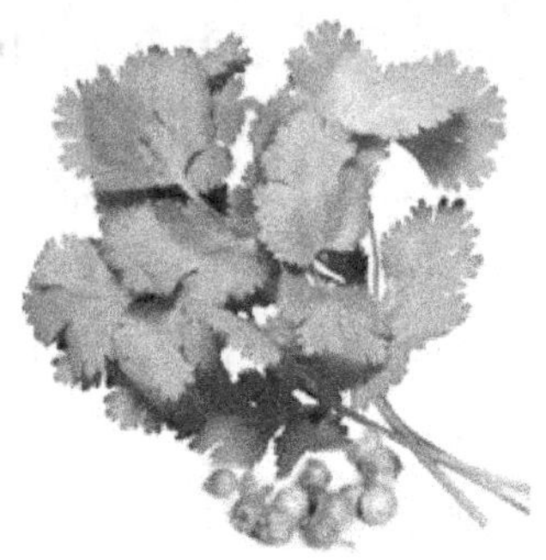

Cumin (*Jeera*)

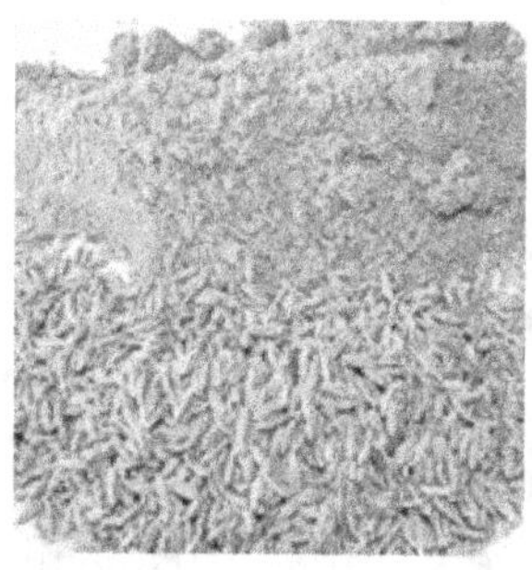

Cumin is pungent, hot, and bitter; it pacifies *vata* and *kapha* and in excess increases *pitta*. Its postdigestive effect is pungent. It regulates digestive function, improving the digestion and absorption and it is used in diarrhea and dysentery. It is also considered beneficial in eliminating bad body odor. It exists in two forms: black (*kala jeera*) and white (*safed jeera*). The aromatic seeds are widely used in Indian cuisine. It is the base of many different kinds of *masalas* used in Indian cooking. It is used in roasted, fried, or powder form.

Asafetida (*Hing*)

Pungent, bitter, hot, and with sulfurous odor, it balances *vata* and *kapha* and increases *pitta*. Asafetida is considered as one of the digestive but powerful stimulants and used in very small quantities. It strengthens intestinal fluid, increases *Agni*, helps in the elimination of gases and destroys round and thread worms. It is used in case of constipation, indigestion, flatulence, abdominal distension, intestinal pain, parasites, arthritis, whooping cough, asthma, epilepsy, convulsions, hysteria, and throbs. It is advised for nursing mothers since it purifies and increases the milk.  Used in Indian households to boil the legumes with a pinch of asafetida to neutralize the gas-producing effect.

Nutmeg

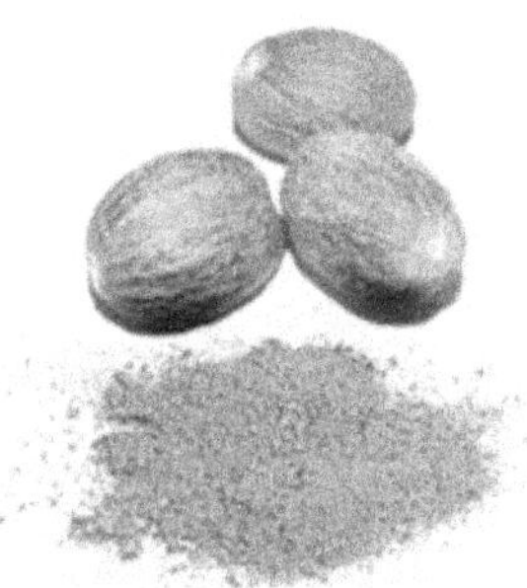 Nutmeg is pungent, bitter, and astringent, and hot and has pungent postdigestive effect. It balances *vata* and *kapha* but increases *pitta*. It is one of the best spices that improve intestinal absorption and helps in the treatment of diarrhea and dysentery. It is good to calm the mind and to induce sound sleep if taken with boiled in milk before going to bed. When taken in excess, it makes the mind dull. It is also useful in abdominal pain, intestinal gas, nervous disorders, insomnia, impotence, and *ama* in the colon. It is suitable in urinary incontinence and premature ejaculation and alleviates abdominal muscular spasms.

Cinnamon

It is pungent, sweet, and astringent; it has hot and sweet postdigestive effect. It pacifies *vata* and *kapha* without increasing *pitta* if it is not used in excess. It promotes digestion and is carminative. Its aromatic oil is used in toothaches, migraines, and impotence. It is very effective in improving the circulation; it acts as a good expectorant in cold and bronchitis. It helps absorption of complex herbal 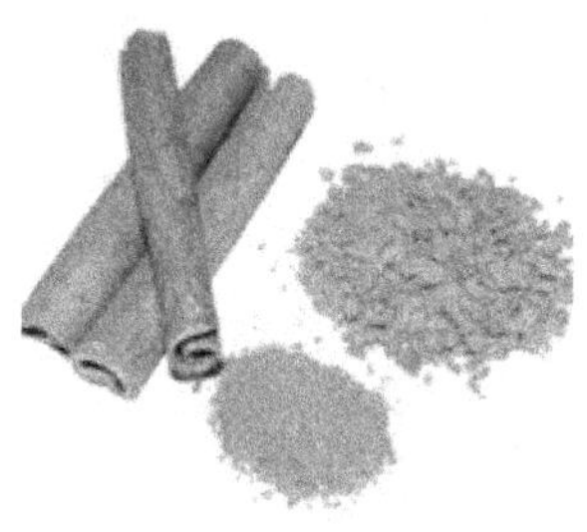 formulas. It is used in kidney conditions and hypertension, being diuretic in nature, helps in urinary disorders. It is used widely in Indian kitchen as one of the main spices for dessert and curries.

Fenugreek

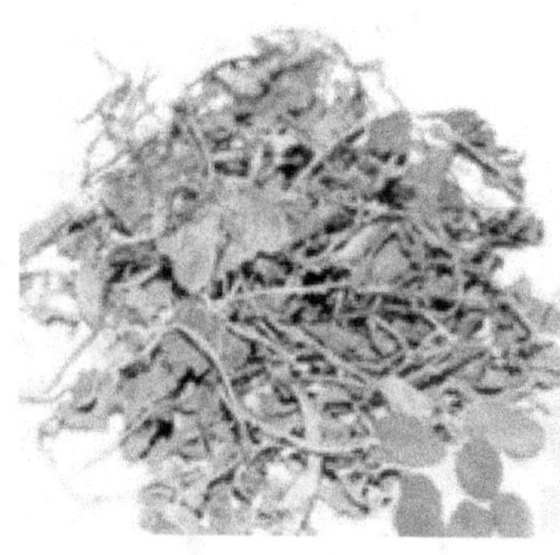 Bitter, pungent, and sweet, it has pungent postdigestive effect; it balances *vata* and *kapha* but increases *pitta* when taken in excess. The seeds improve digestion, alleviate gastric troubles, is carminative and diuretic. The buds of the seeds are used in indigestion, hepatic impairment, and seminal weakness. It is useful in chronic cough, bronchitis, fever, arthritis, and allergies. A paste of fresh leaves applied regularly on the scalp promotes growth of the hair. It increases milk in nursing mothers, because of its high iron content it is beneficial in cases of anemia. It is good for convalescents, mainly for the respiratory system, nervous system, and

reproduction. The leaves are good to cure mouth ulcers. Fenugreek gargles are recommended in throat pains. It is not recommended for pregnant women or high *pitta* conditions.

Basil

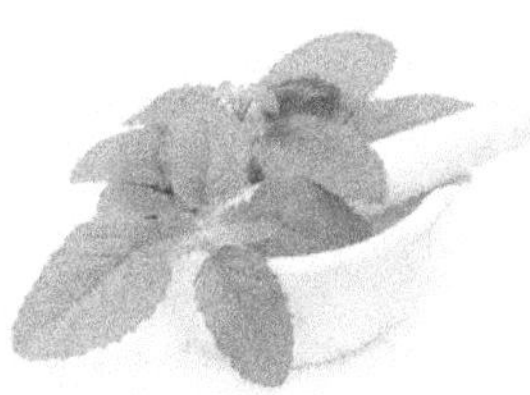

Pungent, astringent, and hot and it has pungent postdigestive effect; it balances *vata* and *kapha* and in excess increases *pitta*. In India, it is considered as a sacred plant and *sattvic*, since it is said that it stimulates devotion feelings, compassion, and faith. In each house one can find a plant of *tulsi* (basil) due to its purifying properties. For a better mental clarity, it can be taken sweetened with honey. In case of skin infections, fresh juice of the leaves can be applied on the affected area. It is used in bronchitis, sinuses congestion, breathing problems, fever, cold and cough, removing excess of *kapha*, and ease breathing. It also removes *vata* when increased in colon, thus improving absorption and abdominal spasms.

Fennel

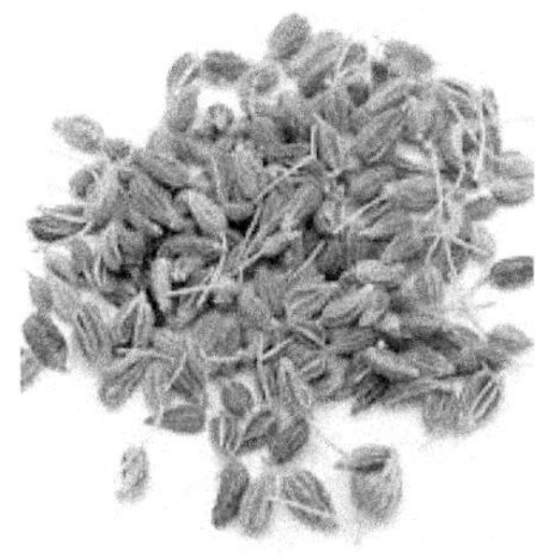

Sweet and pungent, slightly cooling and it has sweet postdigestive effect, it balances all the three *doshas*. The seeds are chewed after the meals to promote digestion and to alleviate gases. Its oil is decongestive and is used in *cough*-related problems. It alleviates premenstrual pain and regularizes menstruation. It increases the flow of maternal milk when taken in form of decoction. It combines well with coriander in urinary problems. It is excellent to stimulate *Agni* without increasing *pitta*, avoids flatulence, and alleviates abdominal spasms. It is also considered as a very good brain tonic.

Saffron

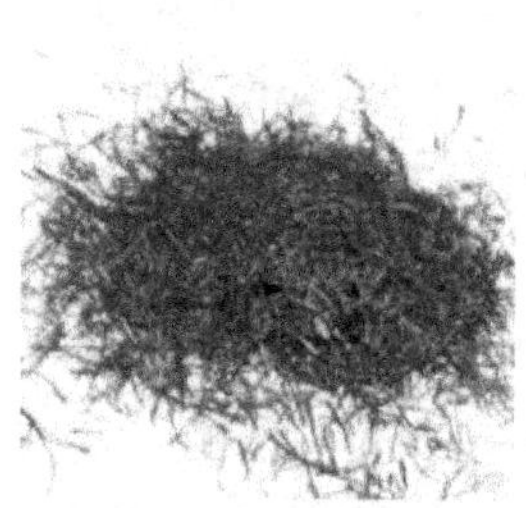

Being pungent, bitter, and sweet, saffron has cold and sweet postdigestive effect. It balances all the three *doshas*. It is used in cases of irregularities or menstrual pain, anemia, menopause, impotence, diarrhea, chronic cough, and asthma. It is considered as an excellent general tonic and a good source of revitalizing the blood circulation and female reproductive system. It is considered as one of the best stimulants, aphrodisiacs, and energizes the subtle body. It is very good to balance *pitta* and regulate the function of spleen and liver.

Mint

Being pungent, slightly cooling, mint has a pungent postdigestive effect. It balances *pitta* and *kapha* but in excess it increases *vata*. It alleviates abdominal spasms, is good for the liver, improves appetite, and acts as carminative. It

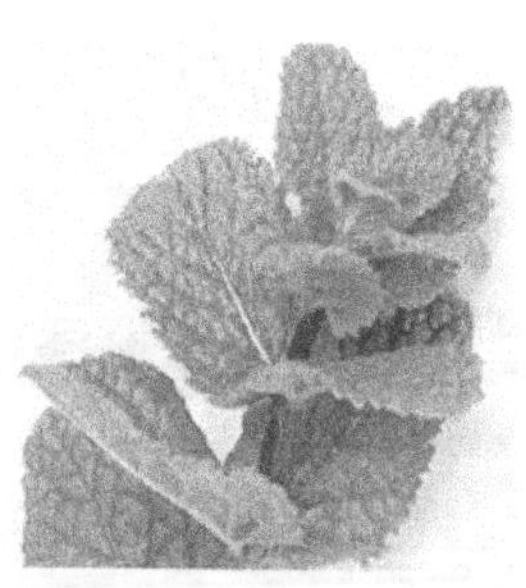

promotes relaxation, mental clarity and helps in emotional tensions and congestion. Gargles with a decoction of mint and salt help cure hoarseness. It is an effective antiseptic mouthwash, strengthens the gums, and prevents the cavity. It is also useful in cold, earache, sore throat, fever, headache, and nervous agitation.

Mustard

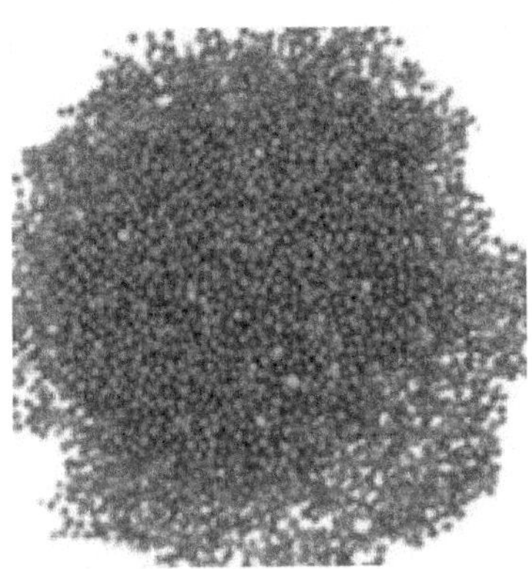

The mustard seeds are pungent and bitter, hot in nature and it has pungent postdigestive effect. It is a strong digestive stimulant for *vata* and *kapha* but can unbalance *pitta* due to its hot properties. In India and abroad, mustard is widely used as a condiment. Mustard seeds are odorless but when soaked in water they emit a very peculiar pungent smell. Mustard oil is widely used in India for cooking, for body, or hair massages. An external application of diluted paste prepared with mustard powder using a lint cloth to avoid burning sensation, it generates heat and serve as analgesic in rheumatism, sciatic, and other muscular pains. Due to its emetic nature, mustard is highly effective in case of poisoning and drunkenness. One spoon of the seeds mixed in a glass of water generally stimulates the vomit after 10 minutes. In case of feverish convulsions in children, a hot water bath mixed with mustard powder can be given for immediate relief.

Cloves

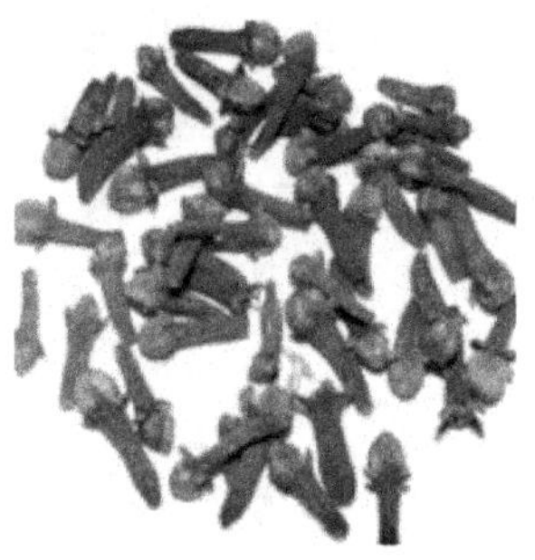

Being pungent, hot, and astringent, the clove has a pungent postdigestive effect. It balances *vata* and *kapha* and increases *pitta*. It contains a volatile oil with strong analgesic effect and is commonly used in India to calm toothache. It is suitable in respiratory problems, cough, asthma, pharyngitis, laryngitis, arterial hypotension, vomits, hiccough, and indigestion. It is carminative, expectorant and disinfects the lymph. It is mildly aphrodisiac and increases blood pressure. It may also cause irritations.

Rose Flower

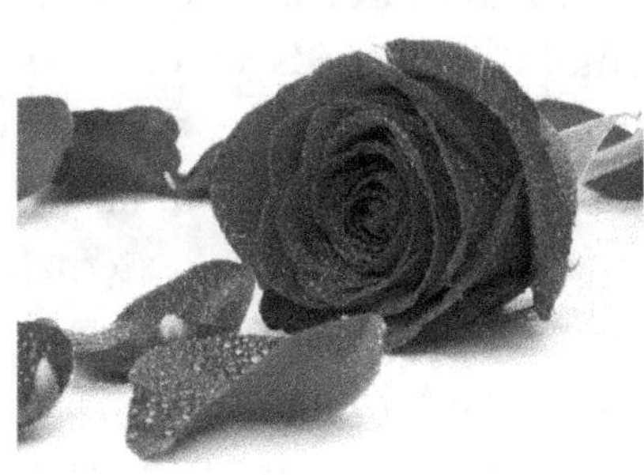

Rose flower is pungent, bitter, sweet, and astringent with a cold. It has a pungent postdigestive effect. It relieves heat and inflammation and is good in reducing *pitta*. It also balances *vata* but increases *kapha* due to its cooling properties. Rose petals are bitter, sweet, and pungent in nature. These are widely used as an eyewash and in the conditions of inflammation in eyes, dizziness, sore throat, headaches, and enlarged tonsils. It is also beneficial for circulatory, nervous, and female reproductive disorders.

Lotus

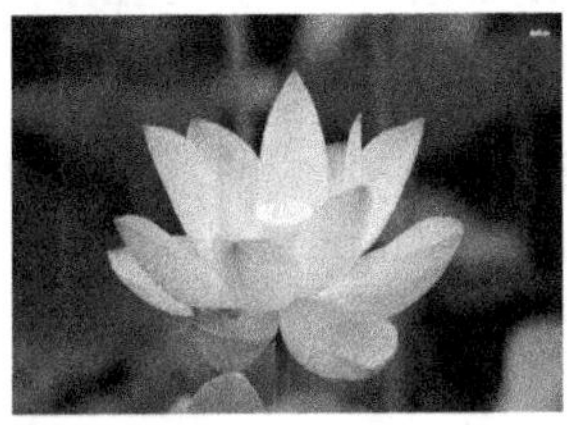

Lotus is sweet, astringent, cold and it has a sweet postdigestive effect. It is a very good *rasayana* (tonic) for heart and reproductive system, decreases *vata*, *pitta*, and increases *kapha*. It is a nutritive and rejuvenative tonic which helps in digestive, circulatory, reproductive, and nervous problems. The root is considered beneficial in blood disorders, hemorrhoids, and diarrhea. It is also considered beneficial in venereal diseases, weak heart, and bleeding disorders.

Ginseng (*Lakshmana*)

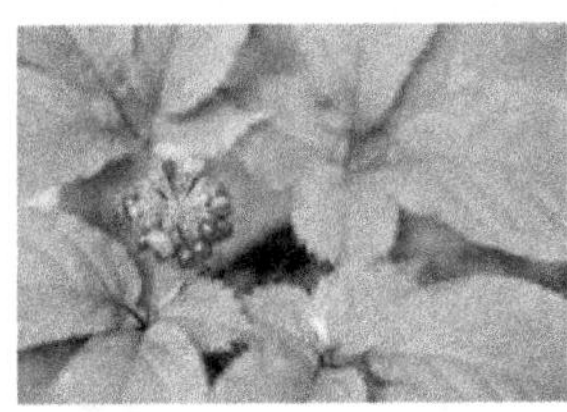

Ginseng is considered as an excellent *sattvic rasayana* for the mind–body complex. Being pungent, bitter, sweet, and hot, it has a sweet postdigestive effect, which makes it useful for all the three *doshas*. It promotes body weight and tissue growth. It is also beneficial in digestive, respiratory, nervous, reproductive, and circulatory disorders. Ginseng is considered as an excellent rejuvenative tonic for old age, debility, fatigue, low energy, and impotence.

Poppy Seeds

Being sweet, pungent, and astringent, poppy seeds balance *vata* and *kapha* and increase *pitta*. These have hot and sweet postdigestive effect. These increase AO (digestive fire), neutralize gas producing in the legumes. Poppy seeds are *tamasic* in nature thus making the mind dull when taken in excess, good sleep inducer and has sedative and analgesic properties. Also beneficial in diarrhea, dysentery, abdominal, and nerve pain.

Ashwagandha (Winter Cherry)

Ashwagandha literally means horse's smell or strength. It is a very powerful *sattvic* tonic for the elderly, debility, and immune system. Being sweet, bitter, and astringent, it has hot and sweet postdigestive effect, balances *vata*, *kapha*, and increases *pitta* when taken in excess. It is considered to be useful for generation of semen, muscle, and nerve rasayana, promotes tissue healing and regenerates hormonal system. It is rejuvenative, aphrodisiac, sedative, and nervine in nature. It is useful in sexual and old age debility, weak eyes, poor memory, paralysis, anemia, infertility, exhaustion, and low energy.

Alfalfa

Being astringent, sweet with cooling, alfalfa has pungent postdigestive effect, mildly cleansing and is detoxifying in nature. It balances *pitta* and *kapha* and increases *vata* when taken in excess. It is a rich source of calcium, magnesium, phosphorus, potassium, and contains all other vitamins. It is helpful in ulcers, vitamin deficiency, arthritis, and mineral deficiency. Being diuretic and hemostatic in nature, alfalfa helps in circulatory and urinary problems.

Jatamansi (Indian Spikenard)

Being sweet, bitter, and astringent with cold, *jatamansi* has pungent postdigestive effect and is an excellent sedative. *Sattvic* in nature, it promotes awareness and sharpens the mind, balances all the *doshas* and is often used combined with other mind-enhancing herbs. It is useful in nervous, digestive, and respiratory problems. It is also helpful in insomnia, epilepsy, migraine, hysteria, convulsions, and tremors.

Brahmi (Gotu Cola)

Being bitter, cooling, and sweet in nature, *brahmi* is one of the important *sattvic* Ayurvedic *rasayana*. It balances all the three *doshas*, is a very good brain tonic and strong blood purifier, promotes longevity and enhances the immune system. It helps in skin disorders, epilepsy, tremors, premature aging, coma, hair loss, nervous disorders, and venereal diseases. It has got the fame of opening and linking the mind to cosmic energy thus attaining name after the god Brahma.

Parsley

Being pungent, bitter, and slightly hot, parsley has pungent postdigestive effect. It balances *vata* and *kapha* and when taken in excess increases *pitta*. Parsley is very rich in minerals, mainly iron and vitamins. It is slightly diuretic, laxative and promotes digestion, dispels kidney and gall stones, alleviates premenstrual pain, and retention of liquid in abdomen and chest. It is also useful in case of edema, swollen glands and breasts, and urinary disorders.

Licorice (Yasthimamadhu)

Licorice is sweet, slightly bitter rhizome, and cooling in nature. It is a tridoshic root, balances *vata*, *pitta*, and amazingly reduces *kapha*. It acts as an expectorant in case of a cold, cough bronchitis, laryngitis, and throat pains. It is beneficial in throat infections and improves the voice. It inhibits inflammation especially in ulcer and gastritis due to a similar active principle of the cortisone. It is a soft laxative that alleviates muscular spasms and reduces inflammation. A high dose of licorice acts as an emetic. Care should be taken as in cases of hypertension and osteoporosis. It reduces the absorption of calcium and potassium.

Pippali (Long Pepper)

Pippali is pungent, hot and it has sweet in postdigestive effect. It balances *vata* and *kapha* and increases *pitta*. It is one of the components of *trikatu*. It is a good stimulant for breathing and digestive system, cures the congestion, and reduces *ama*. It is used in diarrhea, fever, bronchitis, cough, and in stimulating the uterine contraction during the childbirth. It is used as anthelmintic, carminative, and in case of rheumatism. Given in the form of decoctions prepared with milk can help in chronic lung problems as asthma.

Trikatu (Mixture of Ginger, Black Pepper, and Pippali)

It is used to increase *Agni* and burn the toxins of the body. It stimulates appetite and digestion and it is carminative. Its essential oil is secreted by the lungs that reduces discomfort in the pharyngitis and tonsillitis; for that one teaspoon of *trikatu* should be taken with honey. Gargles of *trikatu* decoction are beneficial in dental pains. It is used in powdered form with hot milk for bronchitis. It is also useful in the treatment of congestion sinuses and cold, but as it dries the secretions, it can irritate mucus membranes; for that purpose, it is generally used with *ghee* applied in the nose.

Nuts and Seeds

Nuts and seeds are one of the most important foods since ancient times because of their potential nutrient qualities. They are a rich source of proteins, vitamins, minerals, and carbohydrates needed for human body. Nuts and seeds are often considered as whole foods because of their nutrient rich easily digestible qualities. Most of the vegetarians rely on nuts and seeds for essential proteins since ages. They are also well known for their curative properties. Regular consumption provides resistance against the disease, helps rejuvenating the body, thus preventing premature aging. Today, they are used in various forms in healthy cooking. Sprouted and germinated seeds increase their nutritional value to a great extent. They are also used in the form of oils and butters in cooking as well as in medicine probably due to their high energy and least damaging qualities. They increase the appetite and strengthen digestive tract. There are variety of nuts, the most popular among them are almond, cashew nuts, walnuts, coconut, groundnut, and pistachio; among the seeds are sunflower seed, safflower seed, sesame seed, mustard, etc.

Almonds

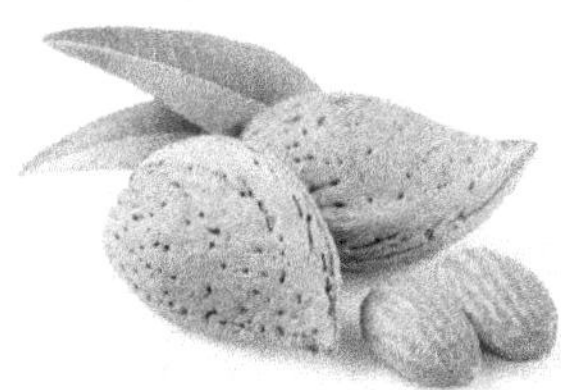

Almonds hold a high esteem among all the nuts, is a highly nutritious food, rich in almost all the elements needed by a human body. It is considered very good for *vata* and *pitta*, whereas for *kapha* it should be taken in moderate amount. It should be soaked for 5 to 6 hours and should be used after removing the thin brown skin by blanching as it is indigestible. Apart from its use in the kitchen, it is widely used in beauty care. Regular application of almond paste with rose buds prevents blackheads, dryness of skin, pimples, and gives a fresh feeling to the face. Almond oil is widely used as a cosmetic product, as well as for dandruff, thinness of the hair, and premature graying of the hair. Almonds are used in curing anemia, constipation, loss of sexual energy, skin diseases, and respiratory disorders.

Coconut

In Hindu mythology, coconut is considered as a tree of health, energy, strength, peace, and long life. In India, the coconut holds an important place in all the religious ceremonies. Being cooling, oily, and heavy, it is extremely good for *pitta*, *vata* people should use it in moderate amount, and *kapha* people should avoid coconut. It is used in various forms in the kitchen as well as in the medicine. Coconut water is quite famous due to its nutrient rich refreshing effects. It is used as dry flakes, in fresh grated form and cubes in rich salads. It

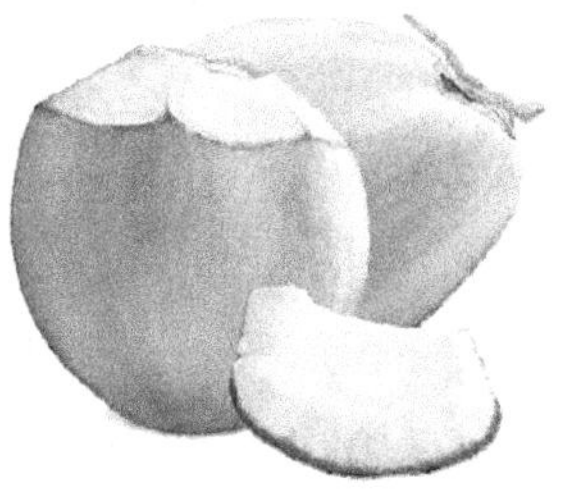

is considered beneficial in the treatment of intestinal worms, digestive disorders, acidity, dry cough, cholera, urinary diseases, and *pitta* and skin disorders. Coconut oil is widely used in the production of cosmetic and eatable products.

Safflower Seeds

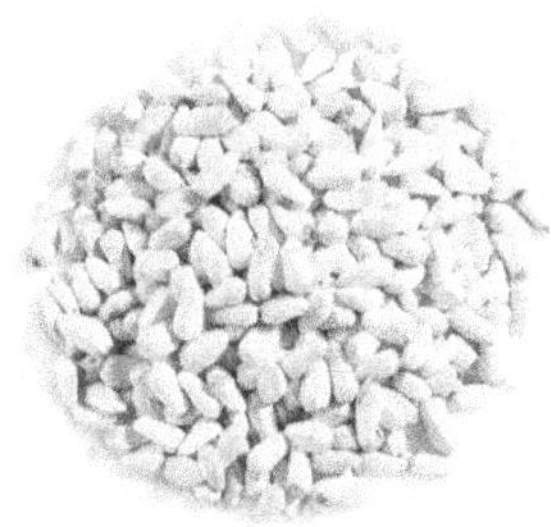

The safflower is an important oil seed crop. It is used mainly in the form of oil in medicine and cooking. It is beneficial for heart problems as it helps lowering blood cholesterol. Being light and dry in nature, it controls *kapha*. The powder of dry seeds is used in curing asthma and respiratory problems, it is also helpful in painful menstruation.

Sesame Seeds

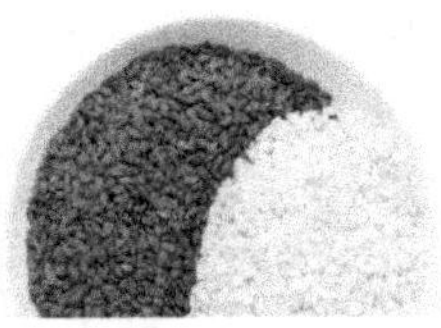

The sesame is a well-known seed crop used all over the world since ancient times especially in Asia. It is available in three main varieties – white, black, and red. The black variety is mainly used for medicines, it also yields the best quality of oil. Today sesame seeds are widely used in cooking due to their high nutritional value and rich in calcium and iron. Sesame oil is considered as the best oil for medicinal use. Its seeds are used to cure piles, skin diseases, respiratory disorders, anemia, painful menstruation, dandruff, and premature graying of the hair.

Sunflower Seeds

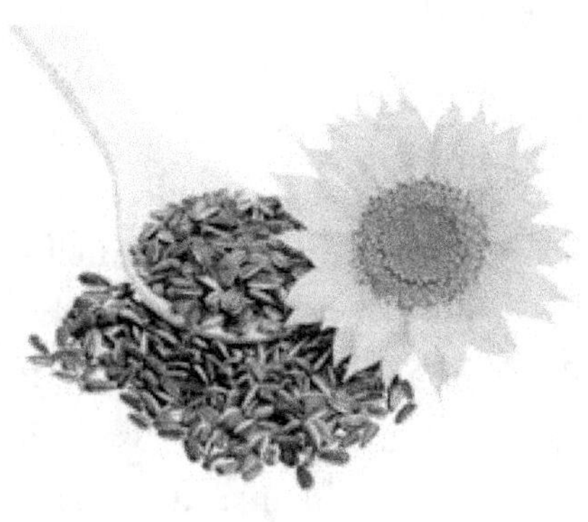

Sunflower seeds are considered as an ideal *kapha* balancing food due to its lightness and easily digestive qualities. It is a rich source of vitamin B complex, proteins, iron, and phosphorus. The seeds control cholesterol level to a great extent. It is also used in the cures of respiratory disorders, anemia, and helps in salt balance in the body. The seeds are widely used in the main dishes, desserts, sauces, chutneys, and soups. The oil gained popularity as an edible oil due to its lightness and low cholesterol level as compared to other oils.

Utensils

One should always use stainless steel utensils for cooking. Glass, porcelain, and wood are also recommendable. One should avoid aluminum and iron utensils as aluminum is a soft metal and during the process of cooking makes the food toxic, on the other hand, iron due to its rusty properties produces toxic effect in the food.

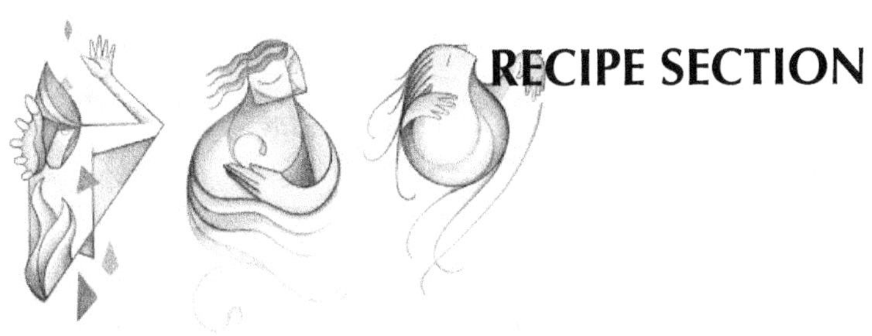

SOUPS

Eggplant Soup

4 Servings   Vata pitta–kapha

Ingredients

2 Cups eggplant   ¼ Teaspoon ground
1 Cup soymilk   pepper
1 Teaspoon corn syrup   Salt and pepper – to taste
¼ Teaspoon oregano   2 Cups water

Preparation

Wash and peel all the eggplants and boil with maple syrup and oregano till tender. Mix in a blender to a smooth consistency using the same water in which it was boiled. Return to fire and add soymilk and the spices. Stir and bring to boil, serve hot garnished with parsley leaves.

Cream of Broccoli Soup

4 Servings   Pitta–kapha

Ingredients

2 Cups broccoli

2 Cups water

2 Cups soymilk

½ Teaspoon cardamom

Salt and pepper – to taste

Preparation

Wash and boil the broccoli, mix in a blender with the same water, add soymilk, check the seasoning and bring to boil stirring continuously. Serve hot.

Sweet Potato Soup

4 Servings

Vata pitta

Ingredients

2 Cups sweet potatoes

2 Cups water

2 Tablespoons corn syrup

2 Cups soymilk

1 Teaspoon fresh ginger

Salt and pepper – to taste

Preparation

Wash the sweet potatoes and boil till well cooked. Peel and blend in a mixer adding water. Return to fire, add spices and soymilk and bring to boil, finally add maple syrup and serve hot.

Pumpkin Shorba

4 Servings

Vata–kapha

Ingredients

2 Cups pumpkin

1 Tablespoon fresh ginger

½ Teaspoon cumin seeds

¼ Teaspoon cinnamon

¼ Teaspoon cardamom

½ Teaspoon coriander or
parsley flakes

Salt and pepper – to taste

3 Cups water

Preparation

Wash, peel, and boil the squash till tender, mix it in a blender with the same water. Chop the ginger, roast the cumin seeds, and powder with a rolling pin. Heat a pan and roast the ginger, add the squash soup, add all the spices and bring to boil. Remove and add roasted cumin powder, stir well, serve hot garnished with chopped coriander or parsley leaves.

Beetroot Soup

4 Servings

Vata–kapha

Ingredients

2 Cups beets (without leaves)

2 Cups water

1 Tablespoon fresh ginger

2 Cups soymilk

Salt and pepper – to taste

Preparation

Wash and peel the beets. Boil them in water until they are soft and pass through a mixer with the same water. Return to fire, add soymilk and season with salt and pepper. Serve hot.

Tomatoes Soup

4 Servings

Vata–kapha

Ingredients

2 Cups diced tomato

3 Cups water

1 Cup soymilk

½ Teaspoon fresh ginger

1 Teaspoon oregano

Clove – a pinch

Asafetida – a pinch

Salt and pepper – to taste

Preparation

Wash and peel tomatoes. Blend with water and then strain everything to remove the seeds. Then put it on low fire along with spices. Finally, add soymilk, boil it for 5 minutes and then remove from heat. Serve hot garnished with chopped parsley leaves.

Cream of Asparagus Soup

4 Servings

Vata pitta

Ingredients

1 Bunch asparagus

2 Cups soymilk

2 Cups water

Salt and pepper – to taste

Preparation

Wash and boil the asparagus, mix in a blender with the same water and strain the mixture through a strainer. Return to fire, add soymilk and check the seasoning. Bring to boil stirring continuously. Serve hot.

Peas Soup

4 Servings

Pitta–kaph

Ingredients

2 Cups fresh peas

2 Cups soymilk

2 Cups water

Asafetida – a pinch

1 Teaspoon turmeric

½ Teaspoon cardamom

Salt and pepper – to taste

Preparation

Boil the peas with water and when they are soft pass through a blender with the same water. Take again to fire, add spices and soymilk. Bring to boil. If dry peas are used, boil for 1 hour adding spices in the beginning.

Mixed Soup Vegetables

4 Servings

Vata pitta–kapha

Ingredients

½ Cup soya beans

½ Cup carrot

½ Cup green beans

½ Cup pumpkin

½ Cup tomato

1 Tablespoon soy sauce

1 Tablespoon vinegar (optional)

Salt and pepper – to taste

Asafetida – a pinch

½ Teaspoon cardamom

Clove – a pinch

½ Teaspoon turmeric

2 Tablespoons brown sugar

1½ Tablespoons cornstarch

3 Cups water

2 Tablespoons sunflower oil

Preparation

Wash the vegetables, peel the squash and carrots, and cut in Julienne. Heat oil, add vegetables, then the spices and stir. Then blend tomato and add water and bring to boil. When the vegetables are soft, add soy sauce and vinegar. In a bowl, mix the corn starch with half a cup of water and add it to the soup stirring frequently. Bring it to boil and serve it hot.

PREPARATIONS WITH *DAL* AND RICE

Pink Lentil *Dal*

4 Servings   Vata pitt

Ingredients

1 Cup pink lentils   ½ Tablespoon ground
1 Unit tomatoes big   chili
2 Tablespoons *ghee*   Asafetida – a pinch
½ Teaspoon cumin seeds   ½ Tablespoon turmeric
1 Tablespoon fresh ginger   Salt – to taste
                                        3 Cups water

Preparation

Soak the lentils overnight. Cook in three cups of water approximately adding salt, asafetida, and turmeric till tender. Wash, peel, and chop the tomato removing the seeds. Heat *ghee* in a pan and put cumin seeds, stir till it turns golden brown, add ginger, chopped tomato, and sweet chili, cook on slow fire stirring frequently till it attains a sauce consistency. Now add this sauce to the cooked lentils. Serve hot garnished with chopped cilantro leaves and a spoon of *ghee* (optional).

RAJMA (Red kidney beans)

4 Servings   Vata pitta

Ingredients

1½ Cup beans red   1 Tablespoon turmeric
1 Head fresh fennel   1½ Teaspoon powdered
2 Medium tomatoes   coriander
2 Tablespoons *ghee*

| ½ Tablespoon ground chili | 1 Tablespoon cilantro leaves |

Preparation

Soak the beans overnight for minimum 12 hours. Cook in eight cups of water adding salt, asafetida, and turmeric till thoroughly cooked stirring occasionally. Peel and chop the tomatoes and the fennel. Heat *ghee* and fry fresh fennel till golden brown, add chopped tomatoes and the spices, cook for 5 minutes stirring well. Add this mixture to the cooked beans. Serve hot garnished with cream and coriander leaves.

Dal De Aduki

| 4 Servings | Vata–kapha |

Ingredients

1½ Cup beans aduki	¼ Teaspoon black pepper
2 Tablespoons corn oil	½ Teaspoon turmeric
¼ Teaspoon cumin seeds	Asafetida – a pinch
1 Teaspoon fresh ginger	1 Teaspoon paprika
¼ Teaspoon clove	Salt – to taste

Preparation

Soak the beans overnight for minimum 12 hours. Cook in six cups of water adding salt, asafetida, and turmeric until cooked stirring occasionally. Peel and chop the tomatoes and the fennel. Heat *ghee* and fry fresh fennel till golden brown, add chopped tomatoes and the spices, cook for 5 minutes stirring well. Add this mixture to the cooked and mashed beans. Serve hot garnished with cream and coriander leaves.

Beans (Mung Dal) Mung Dal

4 Servings   Vata pitta–kapha

Ingredients

1½ Cup beans *mung*   ½ Teaspoon cumin seeds
1 Teaspoon turmeric   Asafetida – a pinch
Salt – to taste   1 Unit tomatoes big
½ Teaspoon ground   1 Teaspoon fresh ginger
pepper   6 Cups water
½ Teaspoon coriander   2 Tablespoons *ghee*/oil
powder

Preparation

Soak the beans overnight. Wash rubbing vigorously in hot running water to remove the husk. Boil adding water, turmeric, asafetida, and salt for 30–45 minutes. Heat the *ghee* or oil and fry the cumin seeds, add one teaspoon of chopped fresh ginger followed by the peeled chopped tomato. Mix powdered coriander and red pepper in half cup of water and add to the tomato mixture. Mix well and cook for 5 minutes or until the *ghee* floats on the surface. Add the sauce to *dal* and check for seasoning. Cook for 5 minutes and serve hot garnished with chopped cilantro/parsley or mint leaves.

Chickpea Dal Chana

4 Servings   Pitta–kapha

Ingredients

1½ Cup chickpeas   2 Medium tomatoes

Asafetida – a pinch
1 Head green fennel
½ Tablespoon turmeric
½ Teaspoon coriander
powder

¼ Teaspoon cumin seeds
¼ Teaspoon ground
pepper
Salt – to taste
6 Cups water

Preparation

Soak the chickpeas overnight in the water. Boil the chickpeas adding asafetida, turmeric, and salt in a pressure cooker for 45 minutes with plenty of water, mash the chickpeas a little with the same water. Chop green fennel and the tomatoes. Heat a pan, roast cumin seeds, add green fennel, stir a while and add tomatoes. Add all the spices and cook for a while and mix this mixture with *chana dal.* Check for seasoning. Garnish with chopped coriander leaves or parsley leaves

Pulao Tridoshico

4 Servings   Vata pitta–kapha

Ingredients

1 Cup rice basmati
2 Tablespoons *ghee*
(optional)
3 Units cloves
3 Units cardamom

3 Units black pepper
3 Units cinnamon sticks
Salt – to taste
2 Cups water

Preparation

Wash the rice, boil the water. Heat *ghee* in a pan and add all the spices, roast till golden brown. Add rice and stir for a while and add hot water and salt, bring to boil, cover and cook on slow fire till all the water evaporates.

Remove from fire and keep the rice covered with the lid for 5 minutes. Serve hot with *dal* or vegetable dish.

Vegetable *Pulao*

4 Servings   Vata pitta–kapha

Ingredients

1 Cup rice

¼ Cup fresh peas

¼ Cup potatoes

¼ Cup carrots

¼ Cup green beans

¼ Cup cauliflower

½ Teaspoon ground chili

5 Units Cardamom whole

5 Units Cloves

3–5 Units Cinnamon sticks

½ Teaspoon Ground cumin seeds

Cilantro leaves for garnish

Salt – to taste

2 Teaspoons *ghee*/oil

2 Cups Water

Preparation

Wash, peel, and cut the potatoes, carrots, green beans, and cauliflower in small cubes. Wash the rice and soak for 15 minutes. Heat the oil or *ghee* in a saucepan and fry the cloves, cumin seeds, cinnamon, and cardamom until golden brown. Add rice and mix with the spices until attains a white color. Add water, salt, and sweet pepper. Now add vegetables and cover the saucepan. Cook until the vegetables are soft and water has been absorbed, leave it covered for 10 minutes. Garnish with chopped cilantro leaves.

Kesari Pulao

4 Servings   Vata pitta

Ingredients

1 Cup rice	3 Tablespoons Brown sugar
6 Units cardamom	¼ Teaspoon *Kesar*/essence of pineapple
4 Units cloves	
4 Units cinnamon sticks	
¼ Cup raisins	1 Cup Water
¼ Cup pistachio nuts	1 Cup Soymilk
¼ Cup almonds peeled	Salt – to taste
¼ Cup cashew kernels	
2 Spoons *ghee*	

Preparation

Wash and soak the rice for 15 minutes. Prepare the syrup mixing sugar and water boiling for 10 minutes. Heat the *ghee* and fry the cinnamon, cloves, and cardamom in a saucepan. Add rice and syrup and cook on slow fire until the water has evaporated. Add milk and *kesar*/pineapple essence stirring occasionally. Cook until all the milk is absorbed. Add raisins, cashew nuts, pistachios, and almonds (peeled), cover the saucepan. Serve hot. *Note:* This *pulao* is sweet and salty in taste.

Tahiri Pulao

4 Servings	Vata pitta

Ingredients

1 Cup rice	½ Teaspoon coriander powder
½ *Taza* potato	
½ *Taza* tomatoes	½ Teaspoon ground pepper
½ Teaspoon cumin seeds	
½ Teaspoon turmeric	

2 Tablespoons lemon juice
Salt – to taste
2 Cups water

¼ *Taza* Coriander leaves
2 Tablespoons *ghee*/oil

Preparation

Wash and soak the rice for 15 minutes. Wash, peel, and cut the potatoes and tomatoes in cubes. Heat the *ghee* and add the cumin seeds until golden brown. Add rice until it is partially white. Now add potato and tomato cubes and stir. Season with coriander, turmeric, powdered pepper, and salt. Add water, stir, and cook on slow fire. Cover the saucepan and cook until the potatoes are soft and the water has evaporated. Remove from the fire and add lemon juice, mix well. Serve hot garnished with chopped cilantro.

Pulao Wild

4 Servings

Vata pitta

Ingredients

¼ Cup Canadian rice
¼ Cup brown rice
½ Cup basmati rice
2 Tablespoons *ghee*
3 Tablespoons raisins
3 Tablespoons cashew nuts

3 Tablespoons walnuts
3 Tablespoons pistachios
¼ Teaspoon powdered cinnamon
½ Teaspoon cardamom
¼ Teaspoon pepper
Salt – to taste

Preparation

Wash each type of rice separate and cook with water and salt in the following proportions:

1 part of rice Basmati – 2 parts of hot water
1 part of integral rice – 4 parts of hot water
1 part of Canadian rice – 2 parts of hot water
Heat *ghee* in a pot and add spices, add raisins, walnuts, cashew nuts, and finally the three types of cooked rice. Mix well and garnish with chopped pistachios.

Spinach With Coconut Rice

4 Servings   Vata pitta

Ingredients

1 Cup basmati rice   3 Units bay leaves
½ Cup spinach   ½ Cup grated coconut
1 Tablespoon fresh ginger   3 Units tomatoes medium
4 Units cinnamon sticks   2 Tablespoons cornstarch
5 Units cardamom seeds   Salt/pepper – to taste
3 Units cloves   Nutmeg – a pinch
½ Teaspoon turmeric

Preparation

Wash spinach and cut finely. Wash rice and keep aside. Heat *ghee* in a pan and add all the whole spices and cook till it turns golden brown, add rice, spinach, and salt, stir and add two cups of the water. Cover and cook till the rice is cooked. In a separate pan boil three cups of water and add grated coconut, finely chopped tomatoes, nutmeg, salt, pepper, and lemon juice. Cook on slow fire for 10 minutes. Meanwhile dissolve cornstarch in half cup of water and add to the coconut mixture stirring frequently till it becomes little thick. Serve hot spinach rice with coconut curry separate or garnished on top.

Simple Khichadi

4 Servings   Vata pitta–kapha

Ingredients

½ Cup basmati rice   ¼ Teaspoon ground
½ Cup mung beans   pepper
½ Teaspoon cumin seeds   Salt – to taste
Asafetida – a pinch   3 Cups water
½ Teaspoon coriander   2 Tablespoons lemon
powder   juice

Preparation

Soak *mung* beans overnight. Wash the rice and beans. In a skillet, roast the cumin seeds, and then add the rice and *mung* beans. Then add all the spices and water, let boil and simmer stirring occasionally. When already cooked, remove from heat. The final consistency should be semiliquid. Check the salt, add lemon juice, stir and serve hot, garnished with chopped coriander leaves.

Ginger Khichadi

4 Servings   Vata pitta–kapha

Ingredients

½ Cup basmati rice   ½ Teaspoon coriander
½ Cup *mung* beans   powder
2 Medium tomatoes   ¼ Teaspoon ground
1 Unit fresh fennel   pepper
1 Tablespoon fresh ginger   Salt – to taste
Asafetida – a pinch   1 Cup water
½ Teaspoon cumin seeds   1 Tablespoon coriander
                             leaves

Preparation

Soak *mung dal* overnight. Wash *dal* and rice thoroughly. Boil rice and *dal* together adding a pinch of asafetida and salt. Peel and chop the tomatoes, ginger, and the fennel bulb separately. Take a sauce pan and roast cumin seeds, add ginger and fennel stirring frequently, when golden brown add the tomatoes, stir for a while and add all the spices. Cook for 5 minutes and add this sauce to the rice and *dal* mixture. Bring to boil stirring slowly. Remove and serve hot garnished with chopped cilantro leaves.

Spinach And Celery *Khichadi*

4 Servings   Vata pitta–kapha

Ingredients

½ Cup basmati rice
½ Cup *mung* beans
Spinach – a bundle
1 Branch of celery
Asafetida – a pinch
½ Teaspoon mustard
seeds

¼ Teaspoon powdered
cloves
Salt and pepper – to taste
2 Tablespoons lemon
juice
4 Cups water

Preparation

Soak the *mung dal* overnight. Wash the rice and *dal* thoroughly. Heat a pan and roast mustard seeds covering with a lid, now add rice and *dal*, stir for a while and add water with all other spices. Bring to boil and cook on slow fire till tender. Meanwhile wash and chop the spinach and the celery. When the mixture is tender add spinach and celery and cook for 5 more minutes stirring occasionally. Check for seasoning. Remove and add lemon juice and serve hot.

Vegetable *Khichadi*

4 Servings   Vata pitta–kapha

Ingredients

½ Cup rice basmati   1 Tablespoon Fresh ginger
½ Cup *mung* beans   ½ Teaspoon Ground
1 Unit carrot   fennel seeds
1 Unit corn   ½ Teaspoon Coriander
1 Unit potato   powder
¼ Cup cauliflower   Asafetida – a pinch
¼ Cup pumpkin   Salt and pepper – to taste
1 Small eggplant   4 Cups water
3 Unit Tomatoes medium

Preparation

Soak *dal* overnight. Wash, peel, and cut all the vegetables into small pieces. Wash the rice and *dal* thoroughly. Take a deep pan and put rice, *dal*, all the vegetables, asafetida, salt, and water. Bring to boil and cook on slow fire till tender. Heat a sauce pan and roast the fennel seeds, add ginger and stir till golden brown, add chopped tomatoes and the spices and cook for five minutes. Now add this sauce to the cooked mixture, check for seasoning, stir and serve hot.

MAIN DISHES

Spinach and Potatoes Masala

4 Servings   Vata pitta–kapha

Ingredients

2 Cups spinach   ½ Teaspoon turmeric
4 Medium potatoes   Salt – to taste
¼ Teaspoon fennel   ½ Teaspoon coriander
powder   powder
Asafetida – a pinch   1 Tablespoon lemon juice

Preparation

Wash and pluck spinach leaves from the stem, wash and boil the potatoes. Boil the spinach in very little water. Peel and cut the potatoes in cubes. Chop boiled spinach. Heat a pan, put coriander powder and stir, add spinach and potatoes immediately. Add fennel, asafetida, and turmeric, salt and lemon juice. Cover and cook for 5–7 minutes on slow fire. Serve hot.

Crispy Eggplant

4 Servings   Pitta–kapha

Ingredients

2 Big eggplants   1 Tablespoon oregano
4 Tablespoons maple   Salt – to taste
syrup

Preparation

Wash and cut the eggplants in slices length wise. Soak in water and salt for half an hour. Place the slices in a tray for oven, sprinkle salt and oregano and pour maple syrup with a tablespoon on each slice. Put little water in the tray, cook in the oven medium hot for half an hour. The water should be absorbed and the borders crispy.

Green Beans In Lemon Sauce

4 Servings   Vata pitta

Ingredients

2 Cups green beans   Salt – to taste
3 Tablespoons lemon   1 Tablespoon cornstarch
juice   ¼ Teaspoon cinnamon
2 Tablespoons fructose

Preparation

Wash and cut the beans in diagonal shape. Boil the beans in little water till tender. Add lemon juice, salt, and fructose, bring to boil. Mix cornstarch in little water and add to the beans stirring frequently. Add cinnamon, stir and cook for 2 minutes, remove and serve hot sweet "n" tangy beans.

Eggplant Rolls

4 Servings   Vata pitta–kapha

Ingredients

4 Medium eggplants   Salt   to taste
1 Tablespoon oregano   ½ Cup water
3 Tablespoons corn syrup

Preparation

Wash the eggplants and cut lengthwise into thin strips. Sprinkle salt and keep aside for 15 minutes. Heat water in a pan, bring to boil and add the eggplants, cook for 5 minutes, remove and cool. Now take the eggplant stripes and roll carefully so that it does not disintegrate. Keep all the rolls in a baking tray, sprinkle salt and oregano. Add maple syrup on top and water, put it in the hot oven for 7–8 minutes.

Eggplant Roasted *Bhurta*

4 Servings   Vata pitta–kapha

Ingredients

3 Medium eggplants   ¼ Teaspoon turmeric
2 Medium tomatoes   Salt – to taste
1 Teaspoon ground ginger   ½ Teaspoon paprika
½ Teaspoon coriander
powder

Preparation

Wash and roast eggplant on direct flame uniformly. Remove from fire and wash off the skin with cold water. Mash the eggplant and keep aside, peel the tomatoes and chop finely. Heat a pan, roast coriander powder, then add chopped tomatoes, salt, ginger, turmeric, and sweet red chili. Cook for 2 minutes stirring frequently.

Now add mashed eggplant. Mix the mixture stirring well. Cover and cook for 5 minutes stirring occasionally. Garnish with coriander or parsley leaves. Serve hot with *dal* and *chapattis*.

Eggplant Roundels

4 Servings   Pitta–kapha

Ingredients

3 Medium eggplants	¼ Teaspoon (*kapha*) black
1 Cup chickpeas flour	pepper
½ Teaspoon coriander	1 Teaspoon fresh ginger
powder	Salt – to taste
¼ Teaspoon ground	Water – as required
pepper	

Preparation

Wash the eggplants, cut into roundels. Sprinkle salt and keep aside for 15 minutes. Wash, peel and chop ginger. Mix chickpea flour, coriander powder, sweet red chili, chopped ginger, and salt. Add water, little at a time to make a batter of a cake consistency. Keep aside for 15 minutes. Wash eggplant roundels and dip in the chickpea batter one by one putting on a hot plate or nonstick pan cooking both the sides till golden brown. Serve hot with any sauce.

Glazed Beets

4 Servings	Vata pitta

Ingredients

2 Cups beetroot	¼ Teaspoon ground
2 Tablespoons maple	cumin
syrup	Salt – to taste
¼ Teaspoon powdered	
ginger	

Preparation

Wash, peel, and slice beetroot, heat one spoon of oil in a pan and add beetroot, stir and add rest of the ingredients. Add water, cover and cook till tender. Remove and serve hot.

Cinnamon Pumpkin

4 Servings   Vata pitta–kapha

Ingredients

2 Cups pumpkin   2 Tablespoons *ghee*
½ Teaspoon fennel seeds   (optional)
1 Teaspoon fresh ginger   2 Cups water
¼ Teaspoon powdered   1 Tablespoon fennel
cinnamon   leaves
½ Teaspoon turmeric
Salt – to taste

Preparation

Wash, peel, and cut the squash into cubes. Heat *ghee* in a pan and roast the fennel seeds till golden brown. Add chopped fresh ginger, stir for a while and add the squash, cinnamon, turmeric, and salt, stir and add water. Cover and cook for 15–20 minutes till the squash is tender. Garnish with fennel leaves and serve hot.

Yoghurt Potatoes

4 Servings   Vata pitta

Ingredients

6 Medium potatoes   ½ Teaspoon ground
1 Cup plain yogurt   pepper
2 Tablespoons *ghee*   ½ Teaspoon turmeric
½ Teaspoon cumin seeds

½ Teaspoon coriander powder

1 Cup water

Salt and pepper – to taste

Preparation

Wash and boil the potatoes. Once cooked peel and cut into cubes. Beat the curd adding water to a smooth consistency. Heat *ghee* in a pan and roast the cumin seeds till golden brown. Add the boiled potatoes and all the spices, stir for a while and add curd. Bring to boil stirring occasionally. Remove from fire and garnish with cilantro or parsley leaves.

Cauliflower For *Kapha*

Kapha

Ingredients

3 Cups cauliflower

1 Large red bell pepper

½ Teaspoon turmeric

½ Teaspoon ground pepper

½ Teaspoon cumin seeds

1 Tablespoon fresh ginger

Salt – to taste

2 Cups water

1 Tablespoon parsley or cilantro leaves

Preparation

Wash and cut cauliflower into florets. Roast the bell pepper on direct fire and remove the skin by putting under running water, cut into small pieces and keep aside. Now roast the cumin seeds in a pan till golden brown and add cauliflower with all the condiments, stir for a while and add water. Bring to boil and cook on slow fire till tender. Remove and garnish with sliced ginger and chopped parsley or cilantro leaves.

Cabbage *Masala*

4 Servings   Kapha

Ingredients

1 Medium cabbage   ½ Teaspoon turmeric
½ Teaspoon cumin seeds   Salt – to taste
½ Teaspoon coriander   Water – as required
powder   2 Tablespoons lemon
½ Teaspoon ground   juice
pepper

Preparation

Wash and cut cabbage in thin strips. Heat a pan and roast cumin seeds till golden brown. Add cabbage and stir, take one cup of water and mix coriander powder, turmeric, and sweet red chili. Add this mixture to the cabbage and stir for a while. Add salt and cook on slow fire till tender. Finally add lemon juice, stir and serve hot with *chapatti* or rice.

Soy Hummus

4 Servings   Vata pitta

Ingredients

1 Cup soya beans   Black pepper – to taste
2 Units red pepper   Asafetida – a pinch
¼ Cup lemon juice   3 Tablespoons fructose
Salt – to taste   2 Sprigs celery

Preparation

Soak soya beans overnight in plenty of water. Remove the skin by rubbing vigorously. Boil soya beans till tender in a pressure cooker. Roast red pepper over the direct flames, remove the burnt skin in water. Put boiled soya beans, red pepper, salt, pepper, celery, fructose, and lemon juice in a blender to obtain a smooth paste. Serve garnished with topping of the choice.

Aloo Mutter (Potato Green Peas)

Vata pitta

Ingredients

6 medium potatoes	Salt – to taste
½ Cup green peas	Black pepper – to taste
1 Unit green fennel	3 Tablespoons lemon
¼ Teaspoon cumin seeds	juice
½ Teaspoon turmeric	Parsley or coriander – for
½ Teaspoon coriander powder	garnish

Preparation

Boil the potatoes with the skin, cool, peel, and cut into small pieces. Wash and chop the green fennel. Heat a pan, roast cumin seeds till golden brown, add coriander powder and chopped fennel, stir for a while. Add boiled potatoes, green peas, turmeric, salt, pepper, and lemon juice and stir well. Add water and boil on a slow fire for 10 minutes. Remove and garnish with chopped parsley or coriander leaves.

Chickpea Masala

Pitta–kapha

Ingredients

1 Cup chickpeas
2 Units potatoes
2 Units tomatoes
¼ Teaspoon cumin seeds
¼ Teaspoon coriander powder
¼ Teaspoon turmeric
¼ Teaspoon ground pepper
Asafetida – a pinch
Salt – to taste
2 Tablespoons lemon juice

Preparation

Soak the chickpeas overnight in water. Boil the chickpeas in pressure cooker adding asafetida, turmeric, and salt till tender, drain off the water. Boil potatoes, peel and cut into small pieces and finely chop the tomato. Heat a pan, roast the cumin seeds, when golden brown add chopped tomato, add all the spices stirring frequently. Add potatoes and chickpeas, stir and cook for 5 minutes. Finally add lemon juice, check for salt, stir and serve hot.

The *Bengali* Vegetables

4 Servings   Vata pitta–kapha

Ingredients

½ Cup carrots
½ Cup green beans
½ Cup pumpkin
2 Units red pepper
½ Cup green peas
1 Cup spinach
1 Head green fennel
1 Teaspoon coriander powder
1 Teaspoon sesame seeds
½ Teaspoon mustard seeds
Salt/pepper – to taste

Preparation

Wash and cut all the vegetables into cubes and chop green fennel. Heat a pan and roast mustard seeds, add green fennel and red pepper, stir for a while and add all the vegetables. Put one cup of water, add sesame seeds, salt and pepper, stir and cover. Cook for 15 minutes, serve hot garnishing with coriander powder.

Vegetable *Uppama*

4 Servings

Vata pitta–kapha

Ingredients

½ Cup semolina

½ Cup carrot

½ Cup green beans

½ Cup cauliflower

1 Unit red pepper

¼ Teaspoon mustard seeds

¼ Teaspoon turmeric

1 Tablespoon lemon juice

1 Tablespoon fresh ginger

¼ Teaspoon black pepper

1 Tablespoon *ghee*

Salt – to taste

4 Cups water

Preparation

Wash all the vegetables, peel and cut the carrots together with green beans in fine stripes. Cut the red pepper in small cube, cut the cauliflower in florets. Heat the *ghee* and add mustard seeds cooking them until they begin to crackle. Add chopped ginger and stir for a while. Add all the vegetables and season with turmeric and salt. Add a cup of water, cover and cook for 10 minutes. Now add the semolina and mix well with the vegetables. Add the three remaining cups of water and cook for 10 minutes more stirring constantly. When the water evaporates add lemon juice. Serve hot garnished with cilantro leaves.

Palak Paneer (Tofu)

4 Servings   Vata pitta–kapha

Ingredients

2 Cup spinach   2 Tablespoons *ghee*
1 Unit fresh fennel   ½ Teaspoon cumin seeds
1 Tablespoon fresh ginger   ½ Teaspoon turmeric
1 Unit green pepper   Salt – to taste
1 Cup tofu/*paneer*

Preparation

Wash and chop the fennel, ginger, and green pepper finely. Wash the spinach leaves and boil with little water (one cup). Once cooked make a puree in the mixer. Cut the tofu/*paneer* in cubes and fry in the pan with half tablespoon of *ghee*. Heat the rest of the *ghee* in a pan and fry the cumin seeds. Add chopped fennel, ginger, and green pepper. Season with turmeric and add the spinach puree. Cook for 5 minutes and check for seasoning. Now add tofu or *paneer* and cook for another 5 minutes on slow fire. Serve hot garnishing with fresh sliced ginger.

Vegetable *Makhani*

4 Servings   Vata pitta

Ingredients

½ Cup green beans   ½ Cup carrot
½ Cup cauliflower   ½ Cup peas

1 Unit fennel
1 Unit tomato
¼ Cup cashews nuts
2 Tablespoons *ghee*/butter
3 Tablespoons sugar
1 Cup water
Salt – to taste

½ Teaspoon ground cumin
½ Teaspoon turmeric
½ Teaspoon ground pepper
½ Teaspoon coriander
1 Teaspoon fresh ginger
1 Teaspoon parsley/coriander

Preparation

Wash and peel carrots and cut in cubes, repeat with green beans. Cut cauliflower in small florets and boil together with peas until they are soft. Peel the tomatoes and take out the seeds, make puree in the mixer, make a paste of ginger and fennel. Heat a spoonful of oil in a pan and fry cumin, then add tomato puree, cook stirring occasionally. When little thick add turmeric, sweet pepper, and coriander. Stir and cook until it thickens. Make a paste of cashew nuts with half cup of water and add to the tomato mixture, cook on slow fire for 10 minutes. Add the vegetables, sugar, and salt to taste and bring to boil. Then add butter or *ghee* followed by cream and serve garnished with cilantro leaves or chopped parsley.

Potatoes Cumin (*Jeera Aloo*)

4 Servings

Vata pitta

Ingredients

6 Medium potatoes
½ Teaspoon cumin seeds

Salt – to taste
½ Teaspoon turmeric

½ Teaspoon ground
pepper

1 Teaspoon cilantro leaves

4 Tablespoons oil/*ghee*

½ Teaspoon coriander

Preparation

Wash and boil the potatoes. When cooked, peel and cut in cubes. Heat the oil in a saucepan and fry the cumin seeds, add spices and potatoes. Add salt and stir, cover the saucepan cooking on slow fire for 5 minutes. Serve garnished with chopped cilantro leaves.

Potatoes Baked With Corn Sauce

4 Servings

Vata pitta–kapha

Ingredients

4 Large potatoes

3 Units fresh corn

½ Cup white flour

2 Tablespoons *ghee*/oil

3 Cups approximately soymilk

Salt and pepper – to taste

¼ Teaspoon nutmeg

Preparation

Wash and dry the potatoes thoroughly and cook in the oven till tender. Meanwhile peel and boil the corns and prepare white sauce, grate the boiled corns and add in the white sauce, add nutmeg and the seasoning and keep aside. Press the cooked potatoes with hands from all sides and make a slit opening on top side. Now pour the hot corn sauce on the potato, garnish with parsley leaves and serve with bread.

Cream of Broccoli

4 Servings

Pitta–kapha

Ingredients

2 Cups broccoli

1 Cup soymilk

2 Tablespoons cornstarch

Salt and pepper – to taste

¼ Teaspoon nutmeg

Preparation

Cut the broccoli into florets and wash. Boil little water and cook broccoli till tender. Remove from fire, drain off the water and add soymilk, bring to boil and add cornstarch dissolved in little water, stir evenly to avoid lumps, add nutmeg and the seasoning and serve hot.

Aloo Gobi

4 Servings

Vata, *pitta*, and *kapha* (occasionally)

Ingredients

2 Medium potatoes

2 Cups cauliflower

¼ Teaspoon cumin seeds

¼ Teaspoon coriander powder

½ Teaspoon turmeric

¼ Teaspoon ground pepper

Salt – to taste

1 Cup water

Fresh ginger – for garnish

2 Tablespoons lemon juice

Preparation

Wash and peel the potatoes and cut into cubes. Cut the cauliflower into florets, wash and keep aside, heat oil in a pan and add potatoes and cauliflower, stir and add all the spices, stir for a while and add water and salt. Cover and cook on slow fire. Remove and garnish with sliced ginger and chopped parsley.

Pickled Green Beans

4 Servings   Vata–kapha

Ingredients

2 Cups green beans   ¼ Teaspoon turmeric
1 Tablespoon fresh ginger   ¼ Teaspoon ground
½ Teaspoon fennel   pepper
¼ Teaspoon coriander   2 Tablespoons oil
powder   Salt – to taste

Preparation

Wash and remove the ends of the beans, boil the beans until partially cooked, drain the water and keep aside. Heat oil in a pan and add fresh ginger, stir till golden brown, add the beans and the spices, cover and cook till done stirring occasionally.

Pancakes

4 Units   Vata pitta

Ingredients

½ Cup white flour   2 Cups soymilk
1 Cup whole wheat flour   ¼ Teaspoon salt*
2 Tablespoons oil

Preparation

Mix the two types of flour and oil with hand until it is very homogeneous. Add soymilk slowly mixing well with a mixer or with hands to make a smooth batter, preferably allow to rest for 1 hour approximately. Heat two to three drops of oil in a frying pan and pour half ladle of the mixture in the pan spreading evenly and thinly, turn upside down. Remove and keep aside.

*in case of salted preparations.

Spinach Cannelloni

6 Units   Vata pitta–kapha

Ingredients

6 Units pancakes   ¼ Teaspoon cardamom
1 Tablespoon oil   3 Tablespoon nuts *
4 Cups spinach*   * sauté in oil for *vata*
3 Tablespoons ricotta   * in *kapha* use reduced
cheese   amounts
Salt and pepper – to taste
Nutmeg – a pinch

Preparation

Wash the spinach and cut the stalks, boil until it is cooked, drain the water chop finely, add salt and pepper to taste and keep aside. Now mix the ricotta with nutmeg and cardamom. Add the chopped nuts and mix with spinach. Put a tablespoonful of stuffing on each pancake and roll or fold in half. Put in the oven for a while and serve hot with the elected sauce.

Seitan

4 Servings   Kapha pitta vata

Ingredients

2 Cups integral flour　　　½ Teaspoon salt
Water – as needed

Preparation

Mix the flour with the salt and prepare a firm dough adding water little by little (as the dough of *chapatti*). Wrap the dough with a humid cloth and allow to rest for half an hour. Put the dough in the disk form in a pan and wash with hot water three to four times eliminating the starch. Cover with water and cook approximately half an hour on slow fire. When it is double in volume, remove from fire. Throw the water and cut in small pieces. Heat oil or butter in a pan and toss it for 5–7 minutes. Serve with preferable sauce according to the constitutional type.

Pasta Dough

Pitta

Ingredients

1 Cup whole wheat flour　　　½ Teaspoon sugar
½ Teaspoon salt　　　½ Cup soymilk

Preparation

To mix the flour, salt, and sugar, sift the flour. Add water gradually mixing with the hand, obtaining a soft dough.

Noodles

Pitta

Ingredients

Pasta dough

2 Liters water

3 Tablespoons oil

Preparation

Sprinkle white flour on the table and roll the dough with the rolling pin according to the preferred thinness of the noodles. Cut with a knife into the long ribbons. Heat the water with oil and when it boils add the noodles. Remove when cooked, strain in a colander and serve hot with the choice of sauce.

Corn Cannelloni

6 Units

Pitta–kapha

Ingredients

6 Units pancakes

2 Units fresh corn

1 Unit red pepper

½ Teaspoon oregano

Salt and pepper – to taste

1 Teaspoon fructose *

1 Tablespoon oil

* avoid for *kapha*

Preparation

Wash and boil the corns, boil red pepper, peel and chop. Grate the boiled corns. Heat the oil and add oregano, then red pepper, salt, pepper and sugar. Cook for 5 minutes and then add the corn. Add half a cup of white sauce. Check the seasoning, put the stuffing in the center of the pancake and fold in the desired shape. Serve hot with the choice of sauce.

BREADS AND SANDWICHES

Integral Wheat Flour Bread

Bread without yeast, oil, or any type of fat.

Mold: 20 × 10 × 5 cm.
Vata pitta–kapha

Ingredients

1 Cup White flour
1 Cup whole wheat flour
1 Tablespoon baking powder

½ Tablespoon salt
3 Tablespoons sugar
Milk soy/water/milk – as required

Preparation

Mix the white flour, whole wheat flour, baking powder, salt, and sugar. Sieve the mixture thoroughly. Grease the mold or use nonstick mold. Add soymilk or water or milk little by little to the mixture until obtaining a batter of semisolid consistency. Beat the batter for 2–3 minutes to add air to the mixture. Pour the batter in the greased mold or in the Teflon mold and put it in the oven (household) on maximum temperature (300 degrees) during 20 minutes and then lower the temperature for 10–15 minutes. To know if the bread is done, insert a wooden stick and if it comes out clean it means that the bread is cooked. Take out of the oven and keep in a cool place for minimum 10 hours before consuming.

NOTE: * You can substitute water for milk or soymilk.
* Not to slice the bread before it has cooled down completely, otherwise bread slices will be moist. To make different types of bread, ingredients can be added to the batter for example: Ginger – 25 grams.

Raisins: 2 ounce/ 50 gram almonds, walnuts or milled chestnuts: 2 ounce/50 grams.

Different spices – anisette/powdered coriander/cinnamon and cardamom – half tablespoon. * You can also sprinkle on the surface of the batter before putting in the oven with Sesame seeds: 1 tablespoon.

Poppy seeds: ½ tablespoon. Kummel seeds: 1 tablespoon.

Chapatti

Vata pitta–kapha

Ingredients

2 Cups whole wheat
(superfine)

Water – as required
Salt (optional)

Preparation

Sift the flour. Add water little by little and knead well to obtain a firm and smooth dough.

Make small balls of 1½ ounce/40 grams each of the dough (dust the balls in the flour every time to avoid sticking of dough to the rolling pin). Roll the balls evenly in the form of disks of 25 millimeter of thickness (approximately) and put on a hot plate. Turn upside down and keep for few seconds and then place directly on the flame moving frequently until it is semitoasted and inflated, turn and do the same. Serve hot, alone or accompanying the main plate applying *ghee* on one side.

Parathas

Vata pitta

Ingredients

2 Cups whole wheat (superfine)

Water – as required

Salt (optional)

2 Teaspoons *ghee*

Preparation

Prepare the same dough as of *chapatti*, make the balls and roll with a rolling pin forming disks. Apply *ghee* on the surface and fold in half, apply *ghee* on folded half and again fold in half forming a triangle. Roll until obtaining the disks in a triangle shape. Place on hot plate and cook both sides applying *ghee* on the surface until golden brown. Serve hot with vegetables.

Note: to make crispy, press with a tablespoon the whole surface while cooking.

Stuffed *Chapatti*

Vata pitta–kapha

Ingredients

For the dough:

2 Cups whole wheat (superfine)

Water as required

Salt – to taste

For the filling:

3 Medium potatoes

½ Teaspoon salt

¼ Teaspoon cardamom

¼ Teaspoon cinnamon

¼ Teaspoon coriander

¼ Teaspoon ground pepper

Preparation

Boil the potatoes and make a puree. Add the spices and mix well. Keep aside. Make the dough as of *chapatti*, make small balls and roll little making a thick disk, put the stuffing with a spoon in the center of the disk, now raise the dough from all the sides and close it pressing the dough making the ball again but with stuffing inside. Now dust the ball and roll out thin into a disk. Care should be taken not to apply too much pressure. Place on the hot plate cooking slightly turning upside down and then place directly on the flame until acquires a golden color.

Apply *ghee* and serve hot with the main foods.

Stuffed Parathas

Vata pitta

Ingredients

For the dough:
2 Cups whole wheat (superfine)
Water – as required
Salt – to taste
For the filling:
3 Medium potatoes

½ Teaspoon salt
¼ Teaspoon cardamom
¼ Teaspoon cinnamon
¼ Teaspoon coriander
¼ Teaspoon ground pepper

Preparation

Carry out the same procedure as for the stuffed *chapatti* but instead of cooking on direct flame it is cooked on the hot plate applying *ghee* or oil on both the sides.

Note: instead of potatoes other vegetables can be used as cauliflower, spinach, cabbage, carrot, grated radish using the same condiments.

Green Pea Patties

Pitta–kapha

Ingredients

1 Cup green peas flour

1 Tablespoon parsley/coriander leaves

1 Unit carrot

¼ Cup green beans

2 Tablespoons raisins

Salt and pepper – to taste

Water – as required

Preparation

Sift the flour of peas, wash and chop well fine parsley or coriander leaves, carrots, green beans, and raisins. Mix all ingredients until batter. Heat a griddle, pour a little oil and add the dough, forming small disks (with the help of a spoon). When it turns up something dry, give it back and cook the other side until golden brown. Serve it hot with a sauce of choice.

Millet Burgers

4 Servings

Kapha pitta

Ingredients

1 Cup millet

2 Tablespoons parsley

2 Tablespoons lemon juice

2 Cups water

Salt – to taste

¼ Teaspoon pepper

½ Teaspoon cinnamon

2 Tablespoons fructose

Preparation

Wash the millet and cook in two cups of water with lemon and spices. Once soft remove from the fire and allow to cool. Add the chopped parsley and fructose, apply oil on the hands and make shape of burgers. Heat oil in a pan and toast the patties from both the sides till golden brown, serve hot with any chutney or sauce.

Potatoes and Corn Burger

4 Servings   Vata pitta

Ingredients

4 Medium potatoes   1 Teaspoon parsley flakes
3 Tablespoons chickpea   ¼ Teaspoon cinnamon
flour   ¼ Teaspoon black pepper
3 Units corn   ¼ Teaspoon coriander
1 Unit red pepper   powder
1 Teaspoon ginger   Salt – to taste
1 Teaspoon fresh fennel

Preparation

Boil, peel and smash the potatoes, grate the corn cob and fresh fennel. Chop red pepper, ginger, and parsley leaves finely. Mix all the ingredients and make small balls pressing slightly to make into the shape of the burgers. Heat *ghee* in a pan and cook both the sides till golden brown. Serve hot with mango chutney.

Soy Milanese

4 Servings   Vata pitta

Ingredients

1 Cup soya beans   Asafetida – a pinch
½ Cup whole wheat flour   Salt, white pepper – to
½ Cup white flour   taste
1 Cup breadcrumbs   6 Tablespoons *ghee*/oil
1 Teaspoon oregano

Preparation

Soak the soya beans for 12 hours, rub them vigorously with hands to take off the skin of the beans, washing and draining the skin that floats on the surface. Put in the mixer and mix well to a paste consistency. Add salt, pepper, asafetida, and oregano and mix well. Add the integral and white flour and make the dough. Make small balls of 30–40 grams and coat with grated bread. Press with the hands to form the disks. Heat 1 tablespoon of *ghee*/oil in a pan and shallow fry the Milanese cooking both sides till golden brown.

Stuffed Milanese

4 Units   Vata pitta

Ingredients

1 Cup Milanese dough   ½ Teaspoon coriander
6 Tablespoons *ghee*/oil   powder
For the filling: Salt – to taste
(1) 4 Medium potatoes   (2) 2 Tablespoons cream
½ Teaspoon ground   cheese
pepper   2 Large tomatoes
                                 2 Units olives

Preparation

(1) Wash and boil the potatoes. Peel and mash with the fork or hands adding the spices.

(2) Wash and peel the tomatoes and take out the seeds. Chop finely the tomatoes and the olives, mash with the cheese and keep aside.

Sprinkle the worktable with the breadcrumbs, make small balls of 30–40 grams/ 1 ounce of the Milanese dough and make flat by pressing with the hand in disk form. Place a tablespoon of stuffing in the center and fold from all sides forming a ball again. Coat with the bread crumbs and press to form the disks. Fry in *ghee*/oil cooking both the sides till golden brown.

Samosas

4 Servings   Vata pitta

Ingredients

For the dough: 2 Medium tomatoes
2 Cups white or whole   ½ Cup Fresh peas
wheat flour   (optional)
8 Tablespoons *ghee*/oil   ½ Teaspoon cumin seeds
Salt – to taste   ½ Teaspoon sweet pepper
Water – as needed   ½ Teaspoon coriander
For the filling: powder
6 Medium potatoes   Salt and pepper – to taste

Preparation

For the dough: Sift the flour with the salt, add melted *ghee* and mix well with the tip of the fingers. Mix with water kneading with the hands until forming a firm dough. Cover with a humid cloth and keep aside.

For the stuffing: Wash and boil the potatoes, peel, and make puree with the hands. Boil the peas and keep aside. Wash, peel, and cut the tomatoes, heat the *ghee*, fry the cumin seeds, and add the tomato and salt. Stir for few minutes and add coriander and sweet pepper. Add the potatoes and the peas and mix well. Remove from the fire and cool.

For the samosas: Make small balls with the dough (30 grams or 1 ounce) and roll thin in form of fine disks. Cut into half and form cone wetting the joints with water. Press well. Stuff the cone with the filling and make a pleat in the superior opening, then seal the borders. Heat *ghee* in a deep pan and fry the samosas until golden brown. Serve hot with tomato sauce.

CHUTNEYS

Carrot Chutney

Ingredients

2 Cups carrots	1 Tablespoon cinnamon
2 Tablespoons fresh ginger	½ Tablespoon cardamom
¼ Cup raisins grapes	½ Cup lemon juice
3 Tablespoons almonds	4 Tablespoons salt
½ Cup sugar	½ Tablespoon pepper
	½ Cup water

Preparation

Wash, scrape, and grate the carrots. Cut the ginger into long strips. Put the carrots and ginger in a deep pan with water and cook on a low fire until tender, add lemon juice, sugar, salt, washed raisins, chopped almonds, and the spices. Cook till it gets little thick in the consistency. Cool and store in clean jars.

Orange And Almond Chutney

Vata pitta

Ingredients

1 Cup orange juice	¼ Teaspoon cinnamon
¼ Cup natural almonds	Salt and pepper – to taste

Preparation

Put all the ingredients in the blender and mix to a smooth paste consistency. Eat fresh.

Lemon Chutney

Vata pitta

Ingredients

2 Cups Lemons	¼ Teaspoon cloves
1 Cup sugar	½ Teaspoon nutmeg
½ Cup fresh ginger	½ Tablespoon pepper
3 Tablespoons salt	

Preparation

Wash the lemons and wipe them dry. Extract the juice and cut long strips of the lemon skin. Boil the lemon in little water till tender with little salt. Put all the ingredients in a pan and cook on a slow fire till it attains the jelly-like consistency. Remove from fire and cool, store in the air-tight jars.

Green Mango Chutney

Vata–kapha

Ingredients

2 Cups green mangoes	2 Tablespoons fresh ginger
1 Cup sugar	1 Tablespoon cardamom

½ Lemon juice cup   1 Tablespoon pepper
4 Tablespoons salt   1 Cup water

Preparation

Wash the mangoes, peel and cut into thin slices. Wash, peel, and chop the ginger. Boil the mango slices with ginger till tender. Now add sugar, salt, lemon juice, and ground spices and cook stirring frequently till the chutney becomes thick. Cool and store in air-tight jars.

Ripe Mangoes Chutney

Vata pitta

Ingredients

2 Cups ripe mangoes   1 Teaspoon cumin
2 Tablespoons fresh   1 Tablespoon ground chili
ginger   ½ Tablespoon pepper
1 Cup sugar   3 Tablespoons salt
½ Cup lemon juice   1 Cup water

Preparation

Wash, peel, and cut the mango in slices, chop the ginger. Blend the mango and ginger with water in a mixer. Put all the ingredients in a pan and cook on a slow fire stirring frequently till the chutney becomes thick. Cool and store in the air-tight jars.

Coconut and Basil Chutney

Vata pitta

Ingredients

½ Cup grated coconut   ½ Cup basil leaves

2 Tablespoons maple or
fructose syrup
¼ Cup nuts

2 Tablespoons lemon
juice
Salt – to taste
1 Cup water

Preparation

Blend all the ingredients in a mixer to a smooth paste consistency. Maple syrup can be replaced by fructose or sugar. Consume fresh.

Basil Chutney

Vata pitta–kapha

Ingredients

1 Cup basil leaves
¼ Cup sunflower seeds
3 Tablespoons lemon
juice

2 Tablespoons fructose
Salt and pepper – to taste
¾ Cup water

Preparation

Roast the sunflower seeds. Wash the basil leaves thoroughly. Put all the ingredients in the blender and mix to a smooth paste consistency. Consume fresh.

Green Chutney

Vata pitta kapha

Ingredients

¼ Cup mint leaves
¼ Cup parsley
¼ Cup fresh coriander

1 Tablespoon fresh ginger
1 Tablespoon lemon juice
Salt and pepper – to taste

Preparation

Separate the leaves of mint, parsley, and coriander. Chop the leaves and put in the mixer with lemon juice, salt, and pepper, mix well making a smooth paste. If the paste is little thick add some water. The flavor is lightly bitter and refreshing. It should be consumed fresh in the day.

Apple and Raisin Chutney

Vata pitta–kapha

Ingredients

2 Large apples

½ Cup raisins (without seeds)

1 Tablespoon lemon juice

1 Teaspoon sugar

Salt – to taste

Nutmeg – a pinch

Preparation

Wash, peel, and slice the apples. Cook them in very little water with sugar and salt. When cooked, put in the mixer with the soaked raisins, the lemon juice and the nutmeg. Mix well to a smooth paste. Return to fire for 5 minutes revolving frequently, if it is very watery, cook until obtaining a semisolid consistency. Allow to cool. This chutney can be conserved in the refrigerator for a month.

Coconut and Parsley Chutney

Vata pitta

Ingredients

¼ Cup grated coconut

1 Cup parsley

2 Tablespoons Maple
syrup

¼ Cup nuts

Salt – to taste

Preparation

Put all the ingredients in the mixer and mix adding some water until obtaining a smooth paste. To be consume fresh.

Kashmiri Mint Chutney

Vata pitta

Ingredients

1 Cup mint leaf

¼ Cup walnuts

¼ Teaspoon turmeric

Salt and pepper – to taste

½ Cup yogurt

Preparation

Separate the leaves of the mint from the stem, wash, and mix with the rest of the ingredients. Pass through the blender until obtaining a smooth paste.

Tomato Chutney

Vata–kapha

Ingredients

4 Medium ripe tomatoes

¼ Teaspoon cumin seeds

¼ Teaspoon coriander powder

¼ Teaspoon turmeric

¼ Teaspoon ground pepper

¼ Teaspoon cinnamon

¼ Teaspoon cardamom

1 Tablespoon sugar

Salt – to taste

1 Tablespoon oil or *ghee*

Preparation

Wash, peel, and cook the tomatoes. Remove from the fire, make a puree and strain. Heat oil in a pan, add the cumin seeds, cook till golden brown. Add the rest of the spices and gradually add the tomato puree. When it boils add salt and sugar and cook on slow fire stirring continuously till it acquires a sauce consistency. Remove off the fire and allow to cool. Store in airtight jars.

Tamarind Chutney

Vata–kapha

Ingredients

½ Cup tamarind pulp
¼ Cup cashew nuts
4 Tablespoons sugar

Salt – to taste
1 Cup water
1 Tablespoon lemon juice

Preparation

Make a paste with the cashew nuts in the mixer. Mix with the rest of the ingredients and cook on slow fire stirring continuously. When the mixture thickens and the sauce acquires shiny texture, remove from the fire and allow to cool. Bottle in air-tight jars.

Orange and Fennel Chutney

Vata–kapha

Ingredients

1 Cup fresh orange juice
1 Teaspoon fennel

¼ Cup almonds
Salt and pepper – to taste

Preparation

Mix all the ingredients in the mixer until obtaining a smooth consistency. To be consumed fresh.

Red Pepper Chutney and Parsley

Vata pitta–kapha

Ingredients

2 Large red bell pepper
2 Tablespoons parsley
4 Tablespoons sunflower seeds

2 Teaspoons maple syrup
½ Teaspoon lemon juice
Salt – to taste

Preparation

Wash the pepper and cut in slices taking out the seeds and boil with little water. Put together with the rest of the ingredients in the mixer and mix well to a smooth paste, using part of the water in which the pepper was cooked. Strain the mixture and put again on the fire until it boils and thicken. It can be conserved in the refrigerator for a week.

Mint and Walnuts Chutney

Vata pitta

Ingredients

1 Cup mint leaves
½ Cup walnuts
4 Tablespoons maple syrup

Salt – to taste
1 Teaspoon lemon juice

Preparation

Wash the mint leaves and toast the nuts. Put all the ingredients in the mixer and mix adding half cup of water until obtaining a sauce. To be consumed fresh.

Dates and Lemon Chutney

Vata pitta

Ingredients

½ Cup dates

2 Tablespoons ginger

2 Tablespoons lemon juice

Salt – to taste

1 Cup water

Preparation

Deseed the dates, peel and chop the ginger and mix in the mixer with the lemon juice and salt, adding one cup of water until obtaining a paste. Put the mixture on the fire and cook for 5 minutes, remove and cool. Store in air-tight jars.

Ginger Chutney and Parsley

Vata pitta–kapha

Ingredients

½ Cup parsley

2 Tablespoons ginger

2 Teaspoons lemon juice

2 Teaspoons maple syrup

Salt – to taste

Preparation

Wash the parsley and chop the leaves. Peel and chop the ginger. Put all the ingredients in the mixer and mix adding three fourth of cup of water until obtaining a soft paste. To be consume fresh.

Walnut and Soy Chutney

Vata pitta

Ingredients

1 Cup soymilk

½ Cup walnuts

2 Teaspoons maple syrup

2 Teaspoons lemon juice

¼ Cup cilantro

1 Tablespoon ginger

2 Pinches nutmeg

Salt – to taste

Preparation

Put all the ingredients in the blender and mix well until obtain a smooth textured sauce.

SAUCES

Mustard Sauce

Vata–kapha

Ingredients

2 Teaspoons mustard powder

1 Cup (approximately) olive oil

3 Teaspoons sugar

1 Teaspoon salt

Pepper – to taste

5 Tablespoons lemon juice

Preparation

Put mustard powder, lemon juice, sugar, and salt in a deep bowl. Mix all the ingredients well and check the flavor. Then add oil gradually to the mixture beating intensely till it becomes thick and shiny.

Mustard Sauce without Oil

Vata–kapha

Ingredients

2 Teaspoons mustard powder
3 Teaspoons sugar
5 Tablespoons lemon juice

1 Teaspoon salt
¾ Cup water
1 Teaspoon cornstarch

Preparation

Put all the ingredients except cornstarch on fire until it boils. Mix the cornstarch with three tablespoons of water and add to mixture on the fire stirring frequently until it thickens. It can be served hot or cold.

Mayonnaise without Egg

Vata pitta

Ingredients

5 Tablespoons soymilk
½ Teaspoon sugar
½ Teaspoon salt
¼ Teaspoon black pepper
¼ Teaspoon mustard powder

A Pinch of turmeric
1 Cup (approximately) corn oil
1 Tablespoon lemon juice

Preparation

Mix the soymilk well with the salt, the sugar, the pepper, the mustard, and the lemon juice. Add the oil little by little stirring frequently until obtaining a thick and shiny sauce. It is recommended to use the blender or electric beater.

Tomato Sauce

Vata–kapha

Ingredients

1 Cup tomatoes

1 Tablespoon sunflower oil

½ Tablespoon oregano

1½ Teaspoons sugar

Salt and pepper – to taste

¼ Cup water

Preparation

Wash, peel, and take out the seeds of the tomato and chop very fine. Heat the oil in a pan, add oregano and stir. Add tomato and season with sugar, salt, and pepper, bring to boil, stir and add 1/4 of cup of water. Cook for 10 minutes on slow fire. Remove when slightly thick.

White Sauce

Pitta–kapha

Ingredients

1 Cup soymilk

2 Tablespoons white flour

2 Tablespoons *ghee*/oil/butter

Salt and pepper – to taste

¼ Teaspoon nutmeg

Preparation

Boil the soymilk and keep aside to cool. Heat the *ghee*/oil and add the flour revolving constantly with a wooden spoon. Care should be taken that the flour should not turn brown. Add the hot milk gradually stirring continuously until acquiring a smooth white sauce. Season and serve hot.

PREPARATIONS WITH YOGURT

Natural Yogurt

Vata pitta

Ingredients

4 Cups milk

½ Cup yogurt

Preparation

Boil the milk and allow to cool. When it is lukewarm, add yogurt or culture, mix well and allow to rest for 12 hours at room temperature.

Dried Fruit Lassi

4 Servings

Vata pitta

Ingredients

2 Cups yogurt

3 Tablespoons almonds

4 Tablespoons sugar

3 Tablespoons pistachios

2 Cups water

½ Teaspoon rose water

Preparation

Add all the ingredients in a mixer and mix well. Decorate with chopped pistachios, serve cold or natural.

Vata Lassi

2 Parts

Vata

Ingredients

1 Cup yogurt

1 Cup water

A Pinch of cumin

Salt – to taste

Preparation

Toast the cumin, blend all ingredients.

Pitta Lassi

3 Parts

Pitta

Ingredients

2 Cups yogurt

1 Cup water

2 Tablespoons sugar

½ Teaspoon rose water

½ Teaspoon cardamom

¼ Teaspoon cinnamon

Preparation

Blend all the ingredients. Serve cold.

Kapha Lassi

3 Parts

Kapha

Ingredients

1 Cup yogurt

2 Cups water

A pinch of black pepper

½ Teaspoon powdered ginger

Nutmeg – to taste

A pinch of cloves

Honey – to taste

Preparation

Blend all the ingredients. Serve at room temperature.

Fruit Lassi

Vata pitta–kapha

Preparation

One can use their imagination and can add different spices and fruits to the lassi: mango, peaches, strawberries, vanilla, banana, etc., respecting the proportions of water and yogurt according to the constitutional type, as well as the fruits or spices advised for each one.

RAITA

Raita is a curd-based accompaniment served with the meals in Indian cuisine. It can be varied using different spices and vegetables according to constitutional type. Its function is to provide the missing flavors in a meal needed by a body.

Eggplant *Raita*

A Cup   Vata pitta–kapha

Ingredients

1 Large eggplant

1 Cup yogurt

¼ Teaspoon coriander

¼ Teaspoon cumin seeds

¼ Teaspoon ground pepper

Salt – to taste

½ Tablespoon mint leaves

Water (if necessary)

Preparation

Roast the eggplant over fire or bake it in an oven until cooked and the skin is burnt. Remove the burnt skin by putting it in the cold water, mash the eggplant and keep aside. Roast and powder the cumin seeds. Now beat the curd to a smooth consistency and add the mashed eggplant and all the spices. Stir it well and garnish with chopped mint leaves. Serve cold with rice or any main dish.

Potato *Raita*

A Cup   Vata pitta

Ingredients
2 Medium sized potatoes   ¼ Teaspoon ground
1 Cup yogurt   pepper
¼ Teaspoon coriander   ¼ Teaspoon cumin seeds
powder   Salt – to taste
                                            Water (if necessary)

Preparation
Boil, peel, and mash the potatoes. Roast and powder the cumin seeds. Beat the curd and add spices and mashed potatoes. Stir well, if thick in consistency add little water. Serve cold with the desired meal.

Carrot and Beetroot *Raita*

Vata   4 Servings

Ingredients
1 Medium carrot   ¼ Teaspoon ground
1 Medium beetroot   pepper
1 Cup yogurt   Salt – to taste
¼ Teaspoon cumin seeds   1 Cup water

Preparation

Wash, peel, and grate the beet and carrot. Roast and powder the cumin seeds. Beat the curd and all the ingredients. Stir and check for the consistency. Serve cold.

Cucumber *Raita*

Pitta   4 Servings

Ingredients

1 Cup plain yogurt   Salt – to taste
½ Cup cucumber   1 Teaspoon mint leaves
½ Teaspoon cumin seeds   (fresh)
¼ Teaspoon black pepper   1 Cup water

Preparation

Peel and grate the cucumber, chop the mint leaves, beat the curd and add all the ingredients. Stir well and cool in refrigerator. Serve with the main dishes as an accompaniment.

DESSERTS

Glazed Pears

1 Serving   Vata pitta–kapha

Ingredients

1 Medium pear   2 Tablespoon maple syrup
Raisin grapes – for
garnish

Preparation

Wash, peel, and slice the pear. Put the slices in hot water for 15 minutes. Decorate the slices on a plate and pour maple syrup on top, garnish with raisins and introduce the plate in the oven for 5 minutes. Serve hot.

Stuffed Figs

4 Servings   Vata pitta

Ingredients

12 Units smirna figs   2 Tablespoons maple
½ Cup walnuts   syrup
12 Units almond

Preparation

Boil the figs until they become slightly soft. Roast the nuts in a pan, mash with the rolling pin, and add the maple syrup. Remove the top end of the boiled figs and open them from the middle with the fingers for stuffing. Stuff with the walnuts mixture. Garnish with a peeled almond on top of each stuffed fig.

Crepe Suzette

4 Servings   Vata–kapha

Ingredients

For the pancake: 2 Tablespoons raisins
½ Cup white flour   For the sauce:
1 Cup soymilk   2 Cups orange juice
Oil/*ghee* (for frying)   4 Teaspoons sugar
2 Tablespoons sugar   ½ Teaspoon cinnamon

Preparation

Mix the flour with oil thoroughly. Add soymilk little by little to make a smooth batter. Heat a pan with very little oil and pour the batter spreading thin. When it leaves the edges turn upside down, cooking on both the sides. Keep aside. Take orange juice in a pan, add sugar and cinnamon and boil until slightly thick. Take the pancake one by one and dip in the hot sauce folding in a triangle, now put the pancake in the center of the plate and add raisins to the sauce, stir for a while and pour the sauce over the pancake. Serve hot.

Delicious Pears

4 Servings   Vata pitta

Ingredients

3 Large pears   ½ Teaspoon cardamom
4 Tablespoons sugar   Raisins (for garnish)
¼ Cup almonds

Preparation

Wash, peel, and cut the pears in cubes and cook them on slow fire with sugar and powdered cardamom. Peel the almonds and put them in the mixer with cooked pears until obtaining a puree. Return to the fire again and cook for five minutes stirring continuously. Check for sugar. Garnish with the raisins, can be served hot or cold.

Coconut Pudding

4 Servings   Pitta

Ingredients

½ Cup grated coconut

1 Cup soymilk

4 Tablespoons sugar

1 Teaspoon cardamom

3 Tablespoons raisins

12 Units almond

2 Tablespoons cornstarch

Preparation

Boil soymilk with cardamom and coconut stirring continuously for 10 minutes. Add sugar and raisins and continue revolving for few minutes. Dissolve corn flour in little water and add to the soymilk stirring frequently and cook until thickens. Allow to cool and garnish with almonds. Serve hot or cold.

Stuffed Apple

4 Servings

Vata pitta

Ingredients

4 Large apples

4 Tablespoons raisins

5 Units dates

4 Tablespoons sugar

½ Teaspoon vanilla essence

Preparation

Wash and peel the apples. Cut into two equal halves and remove the seeds, scoop out the pulp making it hollow for the stuffing. Chop the removed part of the center of the apple and cook sugar, raisins, and chopped dates. Once cooked, stuff the apples with the mixture and put it in the oven with little sugar sprinkled on top till golden brown. Remove and serve hot.

Laddu Chickpea

Vata pitta–kapha

Ingredients

1 Cup flour chickpeas

½ Cup sugar

4 Tablespoons coconut

3 Tablespoons raisins

4 Teaspoons *ghee*

Preparation

Heat the *ghee* and add flour moving constantly until golden brown. Remove from fire and add coconut, raisins, and sugar mixing well until obtaining a homogeneous mixture. Allow to cool a little and make small balls of 1 ounce or 30 grams approximately each with the hands. Store in an airtight jar.

Payasam

4 Servings   Vata pitta–kapha

Ingredients

½ Cup semolina

1 Cup soymilk

3 Tablespoons sugar

3 Tablespoons raisins

3 Tablespoons cashews nuts

½ Teaspoon cardamom

1 Teaspoon *ghee*/oil

Preparation

Heat the *ghee*/oil and add the semolina revolving until it becomes light and white (not golden). Then add the soymilk and the cardamom and cook stirring continuously until the milk is absorbed and the mixture becomes soft. Add sugar and raisins and stir for 5 minutes. Pour in dessert plates and garnish with sliced cashew nuts. Serve hot.

Sweet Potato Pudding

4 Servings   Vata pitta

Ingredients

2 Cups sweet potatoes   ¼ Cup cashew kernels
½ Cup raisins   Grated coconut (to
¼ Cup sugar   garnish)

Preparation

Wash, boil, and peel the sweet potatoes. Mash sweet potato adding sugar. Roughly mash the cashew nuts and add to puree together with the raisins. Grease the molds and sprinkle them with grated coconut. Put in the hot oven for 20 minutes. When the surface turns golden brown remove it from the oven. Remove from the mold turning upside down and serve hot.

Flower of Dates

Vata pitta

Ingredients

For the dough: For the filling:
1 Cup flour   12 Units dates
3 Tablespoons sugar   4 Tablespoons sugar
3 Tablespoons *ghee* or oil   For the sauce:
or butter   ¼ Cup turbinado sugar
3–4 Tablespoons cold   ¼ Teaspoon cardamom
water

Preparation

Take flour and add *ghee* and mix well with the tip of the fingers, add sugar and mix well. Now add water gradually until obtaining a soft dough. Deseed the dates and cut into small pieces, add sugar. Take turbinado sugar in a pan with one cup of water and boil until it thickens, add cardamom and stir well. Roll out the dough evenly and thin and cut into squares. Put one teaspoon of stuffing in the center of the cut square dough, now lift all the four edges and seal pressing them together with the fingers, forming the shape of a small bag. Repeat the process with the rest of the dough. Cook in the slow oven until golden brown. Serve hot with the hot sauce.

Kulfi

Vata pitta

Ingredients

4 Cups whole milk

1 Cup *khoya* (condensed milk)

½ Cup sugar

¼ Cup almonds

3 Teaspoons corn flour

3 Units cardamom whole

¼ Cup pistachio nuts

Preparation

Boil the milk with cardamom. Add *khoya* (condensed milk) and revolve until it thickens. Add chopped pistachios and peeled and chopped almonds. Dissolve the corn flour in little water and add to milk stirring continuously until it thickens. Remove from the fire and allow to cool. Pour the mixture in ice cream molds and put in the freezer overnight.

Dates Souffle

Vata pitta

Ingredients

12 Units dates

3 Cups soybean milk

4 Teaspoons fructose

3 Tablespoons cornstarch

½ Cup water

Preparation

Slit the dates and take out the seed, cut into small pieces and blend in the mixer with soymilk. Put in a pan and bring to boil, add fructose and boil for 5 minutes, dissolve corn flour in water and add to dates stirring frequently, cook for 5 minutes until the mixture becomes thick, remove and pour the mixture in the desired greased molds. Cool and put in the refrigerator for 3–4 hours. Unmold the soufflé and serve cold garnished with chopped dates.

Apple Tart

Vata pitta

Ingredients

For the dough:

½ Cup white flour

½ Cup whole wheat flour

3 Tablespoons fructose

1 Teaspoon baking powder

3 Tablespoons *ghee*/oil

Water (as required)

For the filling:

5 Units apples

5 Tablespoons fructose

3 Tablespoons raisins

Nuts (to decorate)

Almonds (for garnish)

½ Teaspoon cinnamon

Preparation

Wash, peel, and cut the apple into small pieces. Cook on slow fire with fructose, raisins, and cinnamon, when tender add almonds and walnuts. Remove and keep aside to cool. Mix white flour, whole wheat flour, and the baking powder and add oil, rub with the finger tips to mix well, add fructose and add water gradually to make the firm dough. Roll out the dough thin of the size of the tart mold, put the rolled out dough in the greased mold, spread the apple mixture evenly in the mold and cover with another thin rolled dough, prick with a fork in the surface of the dough. Cook in the moderate oven till golden brown. Serve hot or cold.

Apple and Coconut Souffle

Vata pitta

Ingredients

3 Medium apples	2 Cups soymilk
3 Tablespoons coconut grated	6 Tablespoons fructose
3 Tablespoons raisins	3 Tablespoons cornstarch

Preparation

Wash, peel, and grate the apples. Heat the soy milk in a pan, add the grated apple and grated coconut, bring to boil, add fructose and cook for 5 minutes, dissolve the cornstarch in the water and add to the apple mixture stirring frequently till the mixture becomes thick. Pour the mixture in the greased molds and put in the refrigerator to cool for 3–4 hours. Unmold the soufflé and serve cold.

REJUVENATING RECIPES

Dates Milk

Vata pitta

Ingredients

5 Units dates
1 Cup cow milk

A Pinch of cardamom powder
1 Tablespoon honey

Preparation

Soak dates in boiled cow's milk with cardamom powder overnight. Blend the dates with milk and honey in a blender. Drink this date tonic morning and evening. One can increase the amount of dates and milk gradually.

Figs Milk

Vata pitta

Ingredients

3 Unit figs
1 Cup cow milk

1 Tablespoon honey

Preparation

Boil figs in cow's milk, cool and blend in a mixture with honey to a smooth consistency. One can take this milk hot or cold on regular basis.

Buttery Figs

Vata pitta

Ingredients

8 Units figs

½ Cup almonds

1 Tablespoon sugar

1 Tablespoon *ghee*

Preparation

Boil figs for a minute, remove and cut into slices. Soak almonds, peel the skin and chop. Heat *ghee* in a frying pan and add all the ingredients, stir well. Remove and eat hot or cold. It can be accompanied by a hot glass of milk.

Milky Raisins

Vata pitta

Ingredients

¼ Cup raisins black

1 Cup milk

1 Tablespoon sugar

Preparation

Wash raisins thoroughly in lukewarm water. Boil the raisins with milk and sugar. Remove when the raisins are swollen. Eat these raisins followed by the same milk in which they were boiled. The quantity of the raisins should be gradually increased to 50 grams or 2 ounce. This recipe can help in rapid and permanent weight gain.

Bengal Gram Tonic

Vata pitta kapha

Ingredients

2 Tablespoons puffed
bengal gram
5 Dates
5 Almonds

2 Tablespoons milk
powder
1 Tablespoon sugar

Preparation

Make the flour from the puffed Bengal gram. Crush
dates into fine pieces (make powder if dry variety is
available), powder almonds. Add all the ingredients and
mix thoroughly. This mixture should be taken on daily
basis. It makes an excellent dessert, can be eaten alone or
with milk. It can be stored in airtight.

Chickpeas *Kapha*

Kapha

4 Servings

Ingredients

1 Cup Dark chickpeas
2 Tablespoons *ghee*

½ Tablespoon *kapha
churna*
Salt (optional)

Preparation

Leave the chickpeas to soak all night. Drain the water
and add to previously heated *ghee* in a pan. Stir slightly,
cover with a lid and cook at slow heat stirring
occasionally. Then remove from heat and add *kapha*
condiment mix and mix well. It can be served cold or
hot.

Almonds Mix

Vata pitta

Ingredients

10 almonds

1 Tablespoon *ghee*

½ Cup roasted grams

¼ Teaspoon cardamom

½ Cup raisins

2 Tablespoons sugar

Preparation

Blanch almonds by putting in boiling water. Crush roasted grams and chop raisins. Heat *ghee* in a pan and put all the ingredients except sugar, cook for 5 minutes on slow fire stirring frequently. Remove, cool, and add sugar, mix well. Store in air-tight jar.

Tasty Safflower

Vata pitta–kapha   4 Servings

Ingredients

1 Cup safflower seed

½ Cup almonds

¼ Cup pistachio

2 Tablespoons honey

Preparation

Roast and powder safflower seeds, crush blanched almonds, and pistachio nuts. Mix all the ingredients into a fine paste. This mixture should be taken with milk before going to bed.

DIGESTIVE TEAS

Fresh Ginger Tea

Vata pitta kapha

Ingredients

1 Tablespoon fresh ginger   2 Cups water

Method

Wash, peel, and mash the ginger with the help of a rolling pin. Put water on fire with crushed ginger and bring to boil. Boil for 5 minutes, strain and serve hot. *Pitta* should take in moderate amounts with juice of lemon, very good for all the *doshas*, enkindles the *agni* and keeps digestive system healthy.

Dry Ginger Tea

Vata kapha

Ingredients

1 Teaspoon dry ginger powder
2 Cups water

Method

Heat water in a pan and add dry ginger, boil for 5 minutes. Remove from fire and keep for a while, strain and serve hot. *Pitta* should avoid as it is quite heating in nature.

Rose Tea

Pitta

Ingredients

½ Cup rose petals   2 Cups water

Method

Wash rose petals thoroughly, heat the water in a pan with petals and boil for 5–7 minutes. Strain and serve hot or cold. Very refreshing for *pitta* people, also can be used as a face wash in heating conditions.

Cinnamon Tea

Vata pitta

Ingredients

½ Teaspoon cinnamon   2 Cups water
¼ Teaspoon lemon juice

Method

Boil water and add cinnamon, keep it on fire for 5 minutes. Remove, strain, and serve hot. Cools *pitta* and pacifies *vata*.

Licorice Tea

Vata pitta

Ingredients

1 Teaspoon licorice root   ¼ Teaspoon cardamom
powder   1 Teaspoon water

Method

Boil licorice with water for 5–7 minutes. Remove till all the powder settles down, strain and serve hot. Diuretic in action, excellent for *vata* and balances *pitta*, also considered good for hoarse voice and throat problems.

Saffron Tea

Kapha vata

Ingredients

A Pinch of saffron

¼ Teaspoon cloves

A Pinch of black pepper

2 Cups water

1 Teaspoon per cup honey

Method

Heat water and add all the spices, boil for 5 minutes, strain and serve hot with honey. Very good for *kapha* and aids in all respiratory problems, i.e., cold, cough, etc.

Lemon Tea

Pitta vata kapha

Ingredients

1 Unit lemon

2 Cups water

1 Teaspoon per cup honey

Method

Wash and grate the rind of the lemon and squeeze the lemon for the juice. Now add the grated rind and the juice to the water and boil for 5–7 minutes. Remove, strain, and serve with honey.

Mint Tea

Pitta

Ingredients

¼ Cup fresh mint leaves

2 Cups water

Method

Wash the mint leaves thoroughly and boil in 1 liter of water for 5–7 minutes. Remove, strain, and serve hot sweetened with honey in case of *kapha*, a cooling *pitta* tea.

Fennel Tea

Vata pitta kapha

Ingredients

1 Teaspoon fennel seeds   2 Cups water

Method

Add the fennel seeds in water and boil for 5–7 minutes, remove strain and serve hot. It is a very digestive tea for all *doshas*.

GHEE (Purified Butter)

The *ghee* is purified *ghee*/butter/oil. Although it is made with the butter but their properties, according to the Ayurveda, are very different with that of butter in itself. In many cases, the *ghee* is recommended to be used in the diet (in case of having cholesterol, dry skin using internal as well as external). One can prepare the *ghee* using the following recipe:

Recipe: Option One

500 grams or 1 pound Butter

Method

Take a stainless steel pan. Put it on very slow fire with the butter. Let the butter melt and the white melted whey will float on top, remove with the help of a spoon. This process to be continued till the whey is removed completely and the fat part remains at the bottom. Remove from fire, strain, and store in an air-tight jar.

Option Two

500 grams or 1 pound butter

Method

Take the stainless steel pan and put the butter on slow fire. Let the butter boil on slow fire approximately for 25–30 minutes. Keep watching the different stages of the process, the whey will slowly disappear and will form a thin layer so that the fat can be seen clearly. All the whey will stick at the bottom of the pan, at this stage put the fire off without removing the pan. When it cools a bit strain through a muslin cloth or a cotton. Caution should be taken in this process that the *ghee* should not burn. As the fat flows on top and the whey sticks at the bottom, one should put off the fire and the rest will be done from the heat of the stove. To be strained after 10 minutes of putting off the fire.

TIPS TO RELIEVE SOME DISEASES

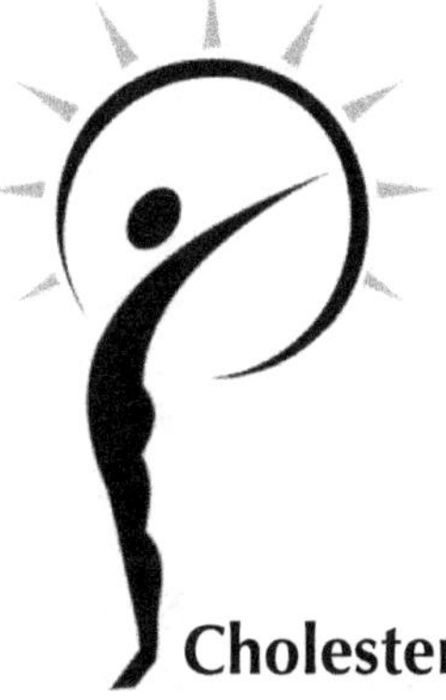

Cholesterol

- o Fresh figs
- o Juice of fresh grapes
- o Grapefruit juice
- o Lemon juice with water
- o Green or raw mango
- o Orange juice
- o Pomegranate juice
- o Amaranth
- o Steamed asparagus
- o Juice or beet salad
- o Karela juice
- o Zucchini juice or prepared as a vegetable
- o Cabbage salad or cooked
- o Carrot juice or cooked
- o Fenugreek leaves or cooked seeds
- o Tea of ginger or cooked in meals
- o Lettuce in juice form or salad leaves
- o Fresh mint juice or prepared as a sauce
- o Chicory Root or leaves in juice or cooked
- o Spinach juice or cooked

o Tomato juice

o Regular consumption of sunflower seeds greatly reduces cholesterol.

Obesity

When it comes to reduce weight we all want to lose it very fast but we fail to understand that all the excess weight was not accumulated overnight. There are various factors that over the period of time account for excess weight, lack of physical activity, overeating, excess intake of sweet and foods loaded with calories, bad digestion, not giving enough of time in between meals so that the food is properly digested. Some of the tips for losing weight are as follows:

o A very effective method for losing weight is an exclusive diet with lemon. The person should begin first day with the juice of three lemons mixed with equal amount of water, drinking it at regular intervals. Every day, it should be increased by a lemon until it reaches 12 and then start reducing the amount of lemons again up to three (day after day). Initially, the person feels weak and hungry, but then he feels normal. This practice is quite hard but very effective. If one feels uncomfortable, he should stop immediately.

o A slow but effective method is to take (on an empty stomach) lemon juice mixed with a glass of hot water and a spoonful of honey daily (for 2 or 3 months accompanied by a low calorie vegetarian diet).

o To lose weight without losing the essential nutrients it is very beneficial to include all the vegetables of leaf, cabbage, spinach, lettuce, chard, etc. in your diet.

o Other way to lose weight is to eat two tomatoes in the morning on empty stomach for 2 or 3 months.

o Take a tablespoon of castor oil mixed with hot ginger tea every morning. This combination removes fat and keeps stomach healthy.

o Drinking hot water with meals is a healthy method, which makes the food digest better and will gradually remove the stored fat.

o In addition to above recipes, a balanced diet that contains all the six flavors in sufficient quantities, combined with regular physical exercise, helps the body to have normal weight.

Cold and Cough

o The daily intake of sweet apples for a week is beneficial in dry cough.

o Another way to cure a cold is to take the juice of one lemon in a glass of hot water, mixed with a teaspoon of honey before going to sleep.

o The hot ginger tea sweetened with honey is good for fighting cold. A teaspoon of ginger juice mixed with honey, three or four times a day, is beneficial for combating cough.

o Onion juice with honey, three or four times a day, helps fight cold or cough.

o Taking a spoonful of the resulting mixture of coconut, seeds of poppy, milk, and honey water, before bedtime, is very beneficial for these disorders.

o The seeds of sunflower or its decoction powder prevent cold.
o Gargling of honey, or consumed directly, immediately relieve cough irritation.
o Gargling of turmeric is beneficial for sore throat.
o A syrup made with the juice of fresh chicory, equal amount of honey and a pinch of salt is very beneficial.
o The mixture formed by a teaspoon of almond oil, a teaspoon of onion juice, and juice of ginger, three or four times a day, is the key to combat whooping cough.

Constipation

o Two raw apples, consumed daily, help regulate bowel movements.
o Damask is a mild laxative.
o Consumption of dates soaked overnight, and then converted into syrup produces a very effective laxative.
o Dried or fresh figs.
o Blending of soaked raisins or grapes juice.
o Lemon juice taken with hot water on an empty stomach.
o Orange juice before going to sleep and fasting.
o Ripe papaya regulates the correct evacuation of the bowels.
o Beets decoction is useful in chronic constipation.
o Raw cabbage in the form of juice or salad.
o Carrot juice mixed with lemon juice and spinach.
o Juice or salad lettuce.

o Tomato juice mixed with salt and pepper (to be taken in the morning).
o Consumption of 10–15 almonds before going to sleep.
o Consumption of seeds of sunflower honey.
o The daily intake of honey maintains healthy stomach.

Diarrhea

o Cooked apples.
o Banana smoothie.
o The paste made from Indian gooseberry leaves mixed with honey.
o Dust from dry seeds of currant of India or an infusion of the leaves.
o Dust from dry seeds with honey mango.
o Pomegranate juice.
o Drinking soup made by boiling the carrot pulp.
o Fresh mint juice mixed with lemon juice and honey (for diarrhea in summer).
o Boiled rice mixed with buttermilk.
o Decoction of Indian chickpeas blacks.
o Coconut with its flesh water.
o Blending of goat's milk, lemon, and toasted peanuts.
o The paste made from roasted sesame seeds mixed with *ghee*, and taken three or four times a day with milk of cow or goat.
o Natural cottage cheese gives immediate relief.

Asthma

o Figs boiled in milk and sweetened with honey.
o Grape juice.

o   A tablespoon of Indian gooseberry (*amla*) mixed with honey.

o   Orange juice sweetened with honey.

o   Juice of Amaranth leaves mixed with honey.

o   A teaspoon of honey mixed with a teaspoon of juice of basil leaves, and a teaspoon of Zucchini paste, at night for a month, before going to sleep.

o   Boil three cloves of crushed garlic in milk, and take every night.

o   Take a clove of garlic, peel, crush, and then boil it in 120 cubic centimeter of pure malt vinegar, then filter it and mix it with equal amounts of honey. Take two or three teaspoons of this preparation with a decoction of fenugreek (every night before going to sleep).

o   Juice of fresh ginger mixed with honey and fenugreek decoction.

o   One part of fresh mint juice mixed with two parts of pure vinegar of Malta, three parts of honey and four parts of carrot juice; mix it well and take it three times a day.

o   A glass of fresh tomato juice mixed with one-fourth teaspoon cardamom powder and honey, before going to sleep, followed by sucking peeled garlic.

o   Half a teaspoon of seeds of safflower powder mixed with honey, two times a day.

o   Milk boiled with turmeric and a pinch of black pepper, sweetened with honey.

Diabetes

o   Drinking the juice of three grapefruit twice a day.

o A tablespoon of juice of Indian gooseberry (*amla*) mixed with a cup of Zucchini juice.

o Infusion of the leaves of mango tree (drink it early in the morning).

o Drink the decoction of fenugreek daily.

o Lettuce in salad or juice form.

o Soybean milk or any preparation made with soybeans.

o Cooked spinach.

o Raw or cooked tomatoes.

o Regular consumption of the black variety of chickpeas.

o The peanuts provide the required nutrients and controlling diabetes.

Anemia

o A good amount of (fresh) apple juice should be taken approximately half an hour before meals and before going to sleep.

o Juice of fresh apricots or consumption of same fruit is very beneficial.

o Daily consumption of bananas.

o The Green mango is also beneficial, and it can be consumed in the form of chutney, *raita* (mixed with yoghurt).

o Raisins have a high content of iron and are very good for this condition.

o Lettuce leaves are considered a good tonic for anemia patients.

o Onions are a rich source of iron and easily assimilate and very beneficial for this condition.

- o The soya beans prepared in light form to be easily digested.
- o Spinach has a high content of iron, so it is highly recommended to be consumed cooked or in juices.
- o Soaked and peeled almonds are useful in this condition.
- o An emulsion of a rate of milk with black sesame seeds.
- o Sunflower seeds flour is one of the richest in iron sources.
- o Honey is very important in the construction of hemoglobin, since it possesses good amounts of iron, copper, and magnesium.

Insomnia

- o Lettuce juice mixed with rose oil is an excellent remedy for massage, in case of mental exhaustion and insomnia.
- o The regular use of lettuce, juice or salad, is an excellent remedy for insomnia.
- o Zucchini juice mixed with sesame oil to be applied on the scalp at night.
- o Cooked zucchini leaves.
- o Head massage with yogurt helps induce sleep.
- o Drink two tablespoons of honey mixed with water, before going to sleep.
- o Boil milk with a pinch of nutmeg and sweetened with honey and walnut.
- o Massage the soles of the feet with milk before you go to sleep.
- o Wash your feet and massage them with sesame oil before going to bed.

Hypertension

- A diet based exclusively on apples gives immediate relief and helps to lower the pressure when it is high.
- Lemon juice and its rind taken as a tea three to four times a day.
- Take two cloves of garlic with water early morning.
- Consumption of cooked brown rice relaxes and calms the nervous system and help to lower the pressure.
- An infusion of licorice root mixed with lemon juice as a tea.
- Any kind of Meditation usually twice a day on regular basis.

Heart Disease

- Consumption of apples because of its high content of potassium and phosphorus and also has low sodium.
- Eating honey at regular intervals.
- Regular consumption of grape juice strengthens the heart. A diet based exclusively on grapes (for 5 or 6 days) provides fast recovery in case of heart pains and palpitations.
- Consumption of the raw Indian gooseberry or in juice form now available in Indian grocery stores.
- The orange juice with honey is a good source of energy, supplying liquid food in heart problems.
- Asparagus juice or steamed strengthens the heart.
- Garlic helps prevent heart attacks.

GLOSSARY

Absorption: healthy acceptance of all the nutrients in the tissues of the body.

Aduki beans: small beans, red, light, and good for strengthening the kidneys; they are very good for *kapha*.

Agni: the sacred fire; It represents all sacred ceremonies in the man's life from birth to death. It is also responsible for the cosmic force of transformation and the digestive fire in the system of human body.

Alterative: purifying and tonic.

AMA: this term is used for the physical, or mental toxins generated by bad digestion.

Amalaki: Indian plant, very rich in vitamin C, also called *amla.* It is widely used in India in medicine because of its healing properties. It is also used in the preparation of *triphala.*

Anabolic: constructive phase of the organism.

Analgesic: effect that relieves the pain.

Aphrodisiac: rejuvenating and toning the body and reproductive organs, invigorating sexual energy.

Aromatic: food or herbs in a strong aroma to stimulate digestion and appetite.

Asafetida: India's strong scent spice that possesses qualities to relieve gas.

Asthi: bone tissue.

Assimilation: the process where the body receives the nutrients.

Astringent: Balancing flavors in *pitta* and *kapha*, due to its refreshing and contractionary properties.

Atharva Veda: one of the four sacred texts of ancient India, known as *Vedas*. It contains the philosophy of Ayurveda.

Basmati: a rice rich in flavor and aroma of Indian origin, known worldwide for providing an easy digestion.

Bhasma: it means ash and is made of burning metals or different medicinal herbs.

Bibhitaki: herb that balances *kapha*, which is also used in the preparation of *triphala*.

Bitter: one of the six essential flavors, cold by nature, good for *pitta* and *kapha*. It cleanses and purifies if used in adequate amounts.

Bloating: unbalanced condition of *vata*, usually with swollen stomach and retention of gas.

Cardamom: an aromatic spice, very popular in the Indian kitchen. Tridoshic by nature, and especially good for *pitta*.

Carminative: which relieves intestinal gas.

Catabolic: the metabolic process of breaking into small particles to improve absorption.

Chana dal: the split form of the black beans, which balance *pitta* and *kapha*.

Chapatti: Indian flat bread, made of whole wheat flour without any preservatives.

Charaka: famous Ayurvédic doctor of ancient India and author of "Charaka Samhita," the classic book of Ayurveda.

Colitis: a condition related to the inflammation of the colon.

Coriander: spice that balances *pitta*, widely used in the cuisine of India. It is good for digestion, and is available in the form of powder, seeds, or green leaves.

Cumin: a digestive spice and tridoshic, very popular in the cuisine of India.

Dal: term used for rich and nutritious soups made from lentils.

Dhatu: one of the seven basic tissues of the body.

Diuretic: eliminate toxins through increase the urine flow.

Dosha: it means unbalance or failure. They are the constitutions of the human body, made of the five elements, *vata*, *pitta*, and *kapha* are called the *doshas*.

Emetic: induces nausea and vomiting.

Emmenagogue: it promotes the menses.

Emollient: soft, tonic. Usually used externally.

Expectorant: it promotes cleansing of phlegm from the lungs and throat.

Fennel: seeds used for cooking and improve digestion. Good for all *doshas*.

Fenugreek: A herb bitter, pungent in nature and something sweet. It is good for *pitta* and *Kapha*. Used in India mainly for making pickles and medicines.

Garam masala: a blend of spices that enhances digestion.

Gastritis: a disease associated with *pitta*, which usually manifests itself with inflammation of the stomach.

Ghee: a purified form of butter, it is made by boiling and clarifying it. It fulfills an important role in Ayurveda and in the kitchens of India.

Ginger: This spice is widely used in the cuisine of India, both fresh and dry. It is also regarded as a great medicine, hot and pungent in nature. It is good for all *doshas*.

Guna: quality.

Haritaki: one of the herbs used to make Ayurvedic medicine called *triphala*.

Hing: see asafetida.

Kapha: dosha or constitution earth–water.

Karma: action.

Khir: Indian dessert made with rice, milk, and shaved with exotic spices. It is eaten hot or cold.

Kichadi: a nutritional preparation made from basmati rice and mung *dal.* It is given to the weak people in order to fortify them.

Bad: waste products from the body, such as urine, feces, and respiration.

Masur dal: red lentils.

Methi: fenugreek greens.

Millet: yellow color which is good for *kapha* cereal.

Mung beans: small green beans, used in the kitchens of India and China. It is available in the diet.

Mung dal: split mung, yellow beans, assorted better digestible and lighter than the latter.

Mustard: Spice, bitter and pungent, available in different colors. It stimulates the digestion and is good for *kapha.*

Ojas: the essential energy of the body.

Panchakarma: literally means the five actions. Also refers to the five cleansing actions of Ayurveda, namely: *basti, nasya, rakta moksha, vamana,* and *virechana.*

Pippali: an Indian variety of the long pepper, which are considered very beneficial to stimulate digestion.

Pitta: a constitution or *dosha* fire–water.

Prana: force or vital energy.

Prasad: sacredly blessed food.

Prithvi: Earth.

Pulao: a dish based on rice and spices, cooked with vegetables.

Rajas: quality of force or energy.

Rajma: a variety of beans, good for *pitta.*

Rakta: blood.

Rakta moksha: an Ayurvedic practice to purify themselves through bleeding.

Rasa: fluid, taste, liquid, feeling.

Rasayana: rejuvenating tonic used in signs of weakness.

Rishis: ancient sages of India.

Sattva: quality of truth, clarity, harmony, peace, and balance.

Sedative: soothing nature.

Saffron: an aromatic spice in a soft yellow color, tridoshico by nature, widely used in Indian desserts.

Sesame Seeds: available in different varieties. Used in the kitchen; its oil is used in therapies with massages.

Shukra: reproductive organs.

Susruta: author of the Ayurvedic text called "Susruta Samhita."

Tamás: quality of inertia.

Tamarind: available in the form of paste or pulp; sour by nature. Improves digestion. Its Indian name is *imli.*

Tofu: soy cheese; good for *pitta*, increases *kapha*.

Tridosha: the three constitutions of the body, namely *vata*, *pitta*, and *kapha*.

Triphala: Ayurvedic medicine used in order to clean and revitalize.

Tulsi: Basil, holy medicinal plant in India. Also used in the kitchen. It is good for all *doshas*.

Turmeric: yellow colored India native spice with antiseptic and antibiotic properties. Widely used in Indian kitchen and as the basis of most of the curries, very good for blood circulation.

Urad dal: small variety of the black beans, which are found in the markets of India.

Vaidya: Ayurveda doctor.

Vata: Constitution or *dosha* air–ether.

Vedas: the four ancient Indian writings, written by hand, containing the knowledge of life.

Vipaka: the postdigestive effect.

Virya: the power of any food substance and its effect, heating apparatus, or refreshing.

BIBLIOGRAPHY

Deepak Chopra, *The Perfect Health*, Bantam.

H.K. Bhakru, *Foods That Heal*, Orient Paperbacks, India.

Robert E. Svobaoda, Prakriti: Your Ayurvedic Constitution, Lotus Press.

R.K. Sharma and Vaidya Bhagwan Das (Trans), *Charaka Samhita*, Volumes I and II (*The Ayurvedic Medical Texts*).

Vasant Lad, *Ayurveda: The Science of Self-Healing*, Lotus Press, Santa Fe, New Mexico.